The
8-Week
Blood Sugar
Diet

The
8-Week
Blood Sugar
Diet

How to Beat Diabetes Fast
(and Stay Off Medication)

Dr. Michael Mosley

ATRIA BOOKS

New York   London   Toronto   Sydney   New Delhi

ATRIA BOOKS

An Imprint of Simon & Schuster, Inc.
1230 Avenue of the Americas
New York, NY 10020

First Atria Books hardcover edition March 2016

ATRIA BOOKS and colophon are trademarks of Simon & Schuster, Inc.

For information about special discounts for bulk purchases, please contact Simon & Schuster Special Sales at 1-866-506-1949 or business@simonandschuster.com.

The Simon & Schuster Speakers Bureau can bring authors to your live event. For more information or to book an event, contact the Simon & Schuster Speakers Bureau at 1-866-248-3049 or visit our website at www.simonspeakers.com.

Interior design by Paul Dippolito

Manufactured in the United States of America

10 9 8 7 6 5 4 3 2 1

Library of Congress Cataloging-in-Publication Data
Names: Mosley, Michael.
Title: The 8-week blood sugar diet : how to beat diabetes fast (and stay off medication) / by Dr. Michael Mosley.
Other titles: Eight-week blood sugar diet
Description: First Atria Books hardcover edition. | New York : Atria Paperback, 2016.
Identifiers: LCCN 2015045485
Subjects: LCSH: Blood sugar—Popular works. | Diabetes—Alternative treatment. | Diabetes—Diet therapy—Recipes. | Diabetes—Nutritional aspects. | BISAC: HEALTH & FITNESS / Diseases / Diabetes. | HEALTH & FITNESS / Healthy Living. | HEALTH & FITNESS / Alternative Therapies.
Classification: LCC QP99.3.B5 M67 2016 | DDC 616.4/620654—dc23 LC record available at http://lccn.loc.gov/2015045485

ISBN 978-1-5011-1122-8
ISBN 978-1-5011-1124-2 (ebook)

To my wife, Clare, for her endless love and support

Contents

Foreword by Dr. Roy Taylor   1

Introduction by Dr. Michael Mosley   5

Section I • The Science

CHAPTER ONE The Obesity Epidemic: Why We're
in the State We're In   17

CHAPTER TWO How Do You Solve a Problem
Like Diabetes?   33

CHAPTER THREE Are You at Risk for Type 2 Diabetes?   55

CHAPTER FOUR Going Low-Carb   65

CHAPTER FIVE The Return of the Very Low-Calorie Diet   79

Section II • The Blood Sugar Diet

CHAPTER SIX The Three Core Principles of the Blood
Sugar Diet and What to Do Before You Start   91

CHAPTER SEVEN The Diet in Practice   115

CHAPTER EIGHT Getting Active   143

CHAPTER NINE Sorting Out Your Head   157

Conclusion   165

The Blood Sugar Diet: 50 Recipes   167

Appendix   227

Acknowledgments   230

Notes   231

Index   237

Foreword

In 2006 I was turning the pages of a scientific journal when one particular page leaped out at me. It was a study of weight loss (bariatric) surgery carried out on obese people with type 2 diabetes. This particular page showed a graph of blood sugar levels following the surgery. Within days of the operation the blood sugar levels had returned to normal and many were able to come off their medication.

This was a striking finding because it was believed that type 2 diabetes was a lifelong, irreversible disease. People are usually advised that they have a condition that requires first pills, then possibly insulin, and they must get used to living with diabetes.

But what really grabbed my attention was the fact that the return to normal blood sugar levels was so rapid. This fit in with a theory I was developing at the time: that type 2 diabetes is simply the result of too much fat in the liver and pancreas interfering with insulin production. The sudden return to normal blood sugars had nothing to do with the surgery itself, but merely that eating had suddenly been cut down. If this theory was right, type 2 diabetes should be able to be completely reversed by food restriction alone.

Science moves slowly and carefully. Any hypothesis has

1

to be tested rigorously. Over the last decade my research team and others working at Newcastle University have been investigating, in detail, the underlying mechanisms. We have developed new ways of measuring fat inside the liver and pancreas using powerful magnetic resonance scanners.

Now we have completed careful studies, which have shown that people who really want to get rid of their type 2 diabetes can, in just 8 weeks, lose substantial amounts of weight and return blood sugar to normal or near normal. They remain free of diabetes provided they keep the weight off. We have shown that it is possible to reverse a disease that is still widely seen as irreversible.

So what is the long-term impact on overall health? Are there drawbacks for some people? To answer these and other important questions Diabetes UK has funded a large study in primary care that will run until 2018.

In the meantime, I am delighted that Dr. Michael Mosley is highlighting the importance of using weight loss to control blood sugar levels. His great skill is in communicating medical science and relating this to everyday life.

In this book about the biggest health problem of our time, he pulls together hard scientific information from reliable sources. He weaves a tapestry that conveys great depth of understanding illustrated by many individual stories. He makes the important point that there is not one diet which suits all, and describes alternatives in a helpful fashion. The relevance of increased daily physical activity as part of long-term avoidance of weight regain is nicely summarized, as is the important interaction between mind and body.

If you have type 2 diabetes and are interested in trying to regain full health, this is a book for you. If the condition runs in your family, then pass the book around the family. In the twenty-first century we individually have to counteract a phenomenon new to our society: for the first time in 200,000 years of homo sapiens' evolution we need to learn how to avoid harm from the ever-present excess of food.

Dr. Roy Taylor
November 2015

Introduction

Millions of us have high blood sugar levels—and many don't know it.

Maybe you're often thirsty or need to urinate frequently. Perhaps you have cuts that are slow to heal or you are unusually tired. Or, far more likely, you have no symptoms at all.

Yet raised blood sugar is very bad news. It speeds up the aging process, leads to type 2 diabetes, and increases your risk of heart disease and stroke.

This is a book about blood sugar. It is about the epidemic of type 2 diabetes that has engulfed the world in recent years. It is also about the insidious buildup of blood sugar that precedes type 2—*pre*diabetes. This is a wake-up call. A warning.

But there's no point in highlighting a problem unless you can do something about it. So if you have type 2 diabetes, I am going to introduce you to a diet that in just eight weeks can reverse it. If you have "prediabetes," I will show you how to stop it from progressing.

Why do I care? Because a few years ago I was diagnosed as a type 2 diabetic, my blood sugar out of control.

First, a bit of background. I trained as a doctor at the Royal Free Hospital in London. After receiving my degree, I pursued a career in journalism, and for the last thirty years I have been making science- and health-related documentaries for BBC Television—first behind the camera, more recently as a presenter. I've reported on many of the great medical issues of the last three decades and interviewed numerous experts on a huge range of topics. This experience has given me a unique perspective. So I'm not exaggerating when I say that the recent rise in diabesity (diabetes plus obesity) is truly scary.

To be honest, for most of my career I was not particularly interested in nutrition. There was next to nothing about the effects of food on the body in my medical training beyond the obvious "eat less, get more exercise," which may be true but by itself is completely unhelpful advice.

A decade ago if you had asked me what I knew about diets, I would have told you with great certainty that the best way to lose weight was gradually, and with a low-fat diet. A pound or two a week was best, because if you went faster you would wreck your metabolism and end up yo-yo dieting. I occasionally tried following my own advice, lost a little weight, then put it straight back on. I didn't realize at the time just how bad my own advice was.

Then three years ago I went to see my doctor and had a routine blood test. A few days later she phoned to say that not only was my cholesterol too high but also my blood sugar was in the diabetic range. I was shocked and wondered what to do, because even then I knew that this is not a trivial disease.

I shouldn't have been surprised. Blood sugar problems are often inherited, and when my father died at the relatively early age of seventy-four he was suffering from a wide range of diseases, including type 2 diabetes, heart failure, prostate cancer, and what I now suspect was early dementia.

Rather than start on a lifetime of medication, I decided to make a documentary for the BBC in which I would seek out alternative ways to improve my health.

While making that documentary, *Eat, Fast, Live Longer,* I came across the work of scientists such as Dr. Mark Mattson at the National Institute on Aging and Dr. Krista Varady at the University of Illinois at Chicago, who were researching something called "intermittent fasting." Years of animal research and numerous human trials have shown the multiple benefits to be had from periodically reducing your calorie intake. These include not only weight loss but improvements in mood and memory.

So I went on what I called the 5:2 diet (eat normally five days a week, cut calories to around 600 on the other two days) and found it surprisingly manageable. I lost 20 pounds in twelve weeks, and my blood sugar levels and cholesterol levels returned to normal. After making the documentary I wrote a book, with Mimi Spencer, called *The FastDiet,* which included not only the science behind intermittent fasting but also a practical guide on how to do it. (For more, visit thefastdiet.co.uk.)

Our book was not aimed at diabetics, however, and I wondered at the time if what had happened to me was unusual. So I decided to look more closely into the science linking calories, carbohydrates, obesity, insulin, and diabetes. That quest has resulted in this book.

Why Now?

Standard nutritional advice is under attack like never before. The age-old instruction to "eat low-fat" has been seriously undermined by numerous studies that show it's rarely effective and people who go on it often find it hard to stick to.

The trouble is that when people cut out fat they get hungry, so they switch to eating cheap and sugary carbs, one of the main causes of the dietary disaster we face today.

And yet, despite everything, the standard advice has barely changed.

For decades governments warned of the dangers of fat while ignoring the dangers of sugary carbs. Many of us know what our cholesterol levels are, but few of us know what our blood sugar is doing, let alone our insulin levels. And we should be concerned, because blood sugar levels are rising at unprecedented rates.

A recent study published in the *British Medical Journal* found that the percentage of people in the United Kingdom who have prediabetes (blood sugar levels that are abnormally high but not yet in the diabetic range) has tripled in the last ten years, up from 11 percent to over 35 percent.[1] And in the United States, according to the Centers for Disease Control (CDC), things are worse: there are at least 29 million people with diabetes, and many don't know they have it. The singer Patti LaBelle discovered she was a type 2 diabetic only when she passed out onstage. Her mother, a diabetic, had her legs amputated, and her uncle went blind from diabetes.

The number of people with prediabetes is even greater. The CDC estimates that it affects 86 million Americans, with fewer than one in ten being aware they are at risk. People of Asian descent are particularly vulnerable; researchers recently estimated that more than 100 million people in that country now have diabetes, while 500 million have prediabetes. Again, most are blissfully unaware.[2]

And prediabetes matters, not just because it normally leads to diabetes but because it is closely linked to metabolic syndrome, sometimes called syndrome X or insulin resistance syndrome. You may or may not have heard of metabolic syndrome, but it is incredibly common—and it is on the rise. Ten years ago I'd never heard of it; now it's everywhere. Metabolic syndrome is also known as the "deadly quartet" because, in addition to raised blood sugar, it includes hypertension, abdominal obesity, and abnormal levels of cholesterol and fat in the blood. Linking them all is the hormone insulin, which you'll be reading a lot more about in this book.

If you have prediabetes (and unless you've been tested you won't know), then there's roughly a 30 percent chance that you will go on to develop diabetes within five years. The actor Tom Hanks was warned by his doctor that he was likely to become a diabetic well before he did, because of persistently high blood sugar levels. Hanks was not particularly overweight. But he was probably carrying too much weight for his particular genetic makeup. (I'll be talking more about "personal fat thresholds" later.) Once you tip from prediabetes into diabetes you will be slapped on medication faster than you can say "Coca-Cola."

In the process of researching this book, I received an email from the daughter of a diabetic. "My mom is embarrassed," she writes. "She thinks it is her fault that she has developed type 2 diabetes. She has always been ashamed of being overweight and yet, despite her best efforts, has never been able to lose the weight. She has not even told my dad (who she lives with!) that she has diabetes, and she only told me because I saw her taking some pills and asked her what they were for." Pills are the obvious answer. But they don't treat the underlying disease, and there are questions about their long-term effectiveness.

Anyway, I'm convinced that there are lots of people who, given the opportunity, would rather get healthy through lifestyle changes than resort to a lifetime on drugs. The tragedy is that they are rarely given the chance. In this book I'm going to make the case for a different and surprising way to combat diabesity and rising blood sugar—and that is to go on a rapid weight loss diet.

"But surely," I hear you say, "that's crash dieting, and crash dieting always fails, doesn't it? You end up putting back on all the weight you lost, and more." Well, no. Like anything, it depends on how it is done. Done badly, a very low-calorie diet will cause misery. Done properly, rapid weight loss is an extremely effective way to shed fat, combat blood sugar problems, and reverse type 2 diabetes.

I am going to take you through the science and demolish many common myths around dieting. And on the way you're going to have to embrace some radical ideas.

I will introduce you to Dr. Roy Taylor, the inspiration for this book. Dr. Taylor is one of Europe's most respected diabetes researchers and he has shown, in several trials, that a very low-calorie diet can, in just a few weeks, do what was once seen as impossible—reverse type 2 diabetes.

You will also meet the people who have used his approach to diet their way back to health: Carlos, a man on the brink of death and who now feels—and looks—twenty years younger. Lorna, who had no idea her blood sugar was out of control, because she was a fit, healthy vegetarian. Geoff, who was about to have a foot amputated, and who wants to save others from going down the same road. Cassie, a nurse who developed type 2 diabetes when she was just twenty-four. After beginning on insulin, she, like many others who start taking medication, put on lots of weight, so much so that she was recently offered weight loss surgery. By following the diet outlined in this book, she lost 45 pounds in two months. She is no longer taking medication and has never felt better. And there's my friend Dick, who also lost about 45 pounds in eight weeks and reversed his blood sugar problems while still enjoying his food and drink. A year later, he is in the best shape I've seen him in for a long time.

These people are not exceptional. Despite being told by their doctors, "It won't work and you'll never stick to it," hundreds of others have done the same.

After losing weight, the real challenge, of course, is to

The Blood Sugar Diet

★ A short, sharp, and effective solution to blood sugar problems

★ Based on scientific trials

★ A clear, precise eight-week plan

★ Inspiring stories of other people's success

★ Advice on what to do after you've lost the weight

keep it off. I will give you clear guidance on the changes you'll need to make to ensure your weight remains steady.

So, do you want to lose weight, improve your health, and get your blood sugar under control? Do you want to achieve this while eating tasty, wholesome food? Well, you're in the right place.

In the next few chapters I'm going to explain why blood sugar matters and what happens if you don't do something about it. But first I want to tell you about Jon.

"I've Found a Way to Live and to Eat"

Jon remembers the moment when he first heard he had type 2 diabetes. It was March 17, 2012. The graphic designer, a forty-nine-year-old father of two teenage sons, was busy with work. His phone rang; it was his doctor's receptionist. "You need to come in right away. Do you feel okay?" she asked anxiously. "Is there someone there with you?"

"I think they were worried I was about to go into a coma," Jon says. Like many people with this condition, he had no idea that he had a problem. Yet his recent test had shown that his blood sugar levels were more than three times the limit of what is considered normal.

People in Jon's age group are developing type 2 diabetes faster than ever before, edging out adults over sixty-five, the group that's traditionally been linked with blood sugar problems.

Jon was put on medication and sent off to talk to nutritionists and dieticians. What followed was months of conflicting advice. One "expert" told him to eat a whole pineapple every day. Another recommended cereal every morning. No one suggested cutting back his calories, despite the fact that he weighed 294 pounds.

When he heard about the Blood Sugar Diet he was immediately interested. It made sense. He liked the fact that it got quick results. He liked the simplicity.

He waited to start until the day after his fiftieth-birthday party. He was hung over. Yet despite feeling terrible, he was ready to begin a new way of eating, which he now says has been "life-changing." He lost 19 pounds in the first week. Let me repeat that—19 pounds. That's how much a car tire weighs. Much of that would have been water, but still, it was impressive.

He was astonished—and immediately motivated to keep

going. For the first time he remembers being able to wear socks and not feel the elastic digging into his swollen ankles. He dropped one jean size in seven days. "It was such a spur," he says, looking back. "I could see right away that this was going to work."

Jon is a warm, funny guy who likes to party. So he fell off the wagon—repeatedly. "I didn't beat myself up," he says. "I'd just start up again the following day. Once I got going, I stopped thinking about it as a diet. I just decided that this is the way I was going to eat." He started walking more and went places by bicycle, further burning up the fat stores.

In three months he lost 50 pounds. Friends and family say he looks twenty years younger. He is no longer on his diabetes medication. His blood sugar results are normal. He uses words like "control," "habit," and "automatic."

"This feels entirely sustainable," he says. "I've found a way to live and to eat."

To eat—and to live. That's what this book is all about.

The Science

CHAPTER ONE

The Obesity Epidemic: Why We're in the State We're In

J ON HAD A SERIOUS WEIGHT PROBLEM, BUT SO, IN-creasingly, does the rest of the world. And this has not crept up on us gradually. People became a bit heavier in the years after World War II, but obesity took off in a spectacular fashion at the beginning of the 1980s; in a single generation it swept the globe.

The fattest people on earth now live in places like Mexico, Egypt, and Saudi Arabia. Countries like China and Vietnam, though still relatively lean, have seen the numbers of overweight adults triple in less than forty years.

Among the rich, developed countries, it is the Americans, British, and Australians who currently lead the pack, with roughly two-thirds of their population overweight.

Men and women in these countries have put on an average of 18 pounds (the equivalent of a large, heavy suitcase) in the last three decades, much of it around the belly area.

Children are particularly at risk. The only type of diabetes that used to be seen in children was type 1, where the immune system mistakenly attacks the cells responsible for blood sugar control. Now many more are coming into doctor's offices with type 2, which is largely due to weight and lifestyle. In the United States, a three-year-old girl who weighed 77 pounds was recently in the news as one of the youngest type 2 diabetics yet seen.

A poor diet affects not just this generation but the next. Overweight mothers are having ever larger babies, who in turn are programmed by the rich diet they get in the womb to become obese in later life.

Obesity spreads like a virus, with family and friends being a major influence on what and how much we eat and what we consider "normal." Being a bit on the chubby side is socially acceptable. There are size 16 models; muffin tops and double chins can be seen everywhere. But while the celebration of curviness has been, in many ways, a desirable response to unrealistically skinny supermodels, it remains a sad fact that too much fat in the wrong places has serious consequences.

So what triggered this explosion?

The obvious answer is that we eat more. In the United States, average calorie intake has increased by over 25 percent since the late 1970s, which would easily account for Americans' weight gain.

But in that same period consumption of saturated fats, such as butter, actually fell. The really big surge, which began in 1980, was in carbohydrates, particularly refined grains, up by a whopping 20 percent in just fifteen years. A study published in the *American Journal of Clinical Nutrition* that compared what Americans have been eating for the last few decades with rates of diabetes could find no link between the disease and the amount of fat and protein consumed.[3] Instead, the researchers blamed the rise of diabesity on falling levels of fiber in the diet, combined with a dramatic rise in the consumption of refined carbohydrates. And what almost everyone now acknowledges is that the rise in consumption of refined carbs came about as an unintended consequence of the war on fat.

The Rise and Rise of Carbohydrates

In 1955 President Eisenhower had a heart attack that nearly killed him. At that time heart disease in the United States was rampant, and so the hugely influential American Heart Association decided, on the basis of what turned out to be rather flimsy evidence, to declare war on saturated fat. Out with steak, butter, full-fat milk, and cheese; in with margarine, vegetable oils, bread, cereals, pasta, rice, and potatoes.

The man who convinced the American Heart Association, and then the rest of the world, to pursue this path was a physiologist named Ancel Keys. In the 1950s he did a study that compared fat consumption and deaths from heart disease in men from six different countries.

He showed that men in the United States, who got a lot of their calories from fat, were far more likely to die from heart disease than men in Japan, who ate little fat. The link seemed clear and compelling. The fact that the Japanese also ate far less sugar and processed foods was discounted. The fact that some countries, such as France, enjoy high rates of fat consumption and yet have low levels of heart disease was dismissed as an anomaly.

The American Heart Association gave Keys its support, and the anti-fat campaign began in earnest. It took a while to get going, but by the 1980s there was a dramatic change in what people were eating all around the world. Huge numbers followed medical advice and switched from eating animal fats, like butter and milk, to eating margarine, low-fat products, and vegetable oils.

The campaign against saturated fat was not just based on fear that it would clog up arteries. Eating fat, it was widely believed, *made you fat*. Ounce for ounce, fat contains more calories than either carbohydrates or protein. So the easiest way to lose weight, it was thought, was to cut down on fat.

Low-fat diets were created and endorsed enthusiastically by the medical profession. My father tried quite a few and lost weight on each. The trouble was, he found them impossible to stick to. He was not alone. The success rate of low-fat diets, even where patients are highly motivated and closely supervised, has been poor.

A poignant example of this was the Look Ahead trial in

2001.[4] Sixteen medical centers in the United States recruited more than five thousand overweight diabetics to take part in a randomized, controlled trial. Half were offered standard care; the other half were put on a low-fat diet. The low-fat group got personal nutritionists, trainers, group support sessions—the best that money could buy.

The trial was due to run until 2016, but it was stopped after ten years because the patients in the low-fat group had lost only a little more weight than the control group and there were no differences in rates of heart disease or stroke. The diabetic patients had managed to cut their fat consumption, but that had not produced either the weight loss or the health benefits that were hoped for.

In the meantime, the campaign against fat was working very successfully, in the sense that the world now ate far more fat-free and reduced-fat "diet" products. But we didn't get slimmer; we became fatter.

Part of the problem was that food manufacturers, when they took out the fat, put in sugar to make their food more palatable. The low-fat Starbucks muffin, for instance (now discontinued, or at least I can no longer find it on the Starbucks website), used to contain 430 calories and the equivalent of 13 teaspoons of sugar. People seemed to think that if a product said "fat-free" on the label, then it wouldn't make you fat. There were doctors telling the public that you can't get fat eating carbohydrates; one leading nutritional expert, Jean Mayer, said that prescribing a carbohydrate-restricted diet to the public was "the equivalent of mass murder."

I started medical school in 1980, when the campaign

against fat was in full flow. I gave up butter, cream, and eggs. I rarely ate red meat and switched to skim milk and low-fat yogurt, neither of which I enjoyed, but both of which I was sure were good for me. Over the next few decades, despite much self-denial, I put on nearly 30 pounds and my blood sugar soared. The high-carb, low-fat diet I was on wasn't making me healthier. It was doing the reverse.

Why?

Carbs and Insulin

Well, the thing about carbs, particularly the easily digestible ones, such as sugar, but also breakfast cereals, pasta, bread, and potatoes, is that they are easily broken down in the gut to release sugar into your system.

Your pancreas responds by producing insulin. One of insulin's main jobs is to bring high blood sugar levels down, and it does this by helping energy-hungry cells, such as those in your muscles, take up the sugar.

Unfortunately, an unhealthful diet and a low-activity lifestyle can, over many years, lead to what's called insulin resistance. Your body becomes less and less sensitive to insulin. Your blood sugar levels creep up. And as they rise, your pancreas responds by pumping out more and more insulin. But it's like shouting at your kids—after a while they stop listening.

While your muscles are becoming insulin-resistant, however, insulin is still able to force surplus calories into your fat cells. The result is that as your insulin levels rise, more and more energy is diverted into fat storage. The higher your insulin levels, the fatter you get.

And yet the more calories you tuck away as fat, the less you have to keep the rest of your body going. It's a bit like buying fuel, but instead of putting it in the gas tank you put it in the trunk of the car. The fuel gauge sinks, but your frantic attempts to top up fail because the fuel is going into the wrong place. Similarly, your muscles, deprived of fuel, tell your brain to eat more. So you do. But because your high insulin levels are encouraging fat storage, you just get fatter while staying hungry.

Dr. Robert Lustig, a renowned pediatric endocrinologist who has treated hundreds of overweight children, points out in his excellent book *Fat Chance* that understanding insulin is crucial to understanding obesity. "There is no fat accumulation without the energy-storage hormone, insulin," he writes. "Insulin shunts sugar to fat. It makes your fat cells grow. The more insulin the more the fat."

He argues that the main reason obesity levels have doubled over the last thirty years is because our bodies are producing far more insulin than ever before. And he blames the modern diet, rich in sugar and refined carbs, for pumping up our insulin levels, a claim supported by many other leading obesity experts, including Dr. David Ludwig, a pediatrician at Harvard Medical School, and Dr. Mark Friedman, head of the Nutrition Science Initiative in San Diego. They recently wrote an opinion piece in the *New York Times* ("Always Hungry? Here's Why") in which they point the finger firmly at refined carbs: "The increasing amount and processing of carbohydrates in the American diet has increased insulin levels, put fat cells into storage overdrive and elicited obesity-promoting biological responses in a large number of people. High consumption of refined carbohydrates—chips, crackers, cakes, soft drinks, sugary breakfast cereals and even white rice and bread—has increased body weights throughout the population."[5]

Dr. Ludwig is worth listening to because for many years he has run one of the largest clinics for overweight children in the United States at the Boston Children's Hospital. He has seen close up how easily digestible carbs (those with a high glycemic load; see page 72) have been a major driver of obesity.

In one study, he took twelve overweight teenage boys and on separate days gave them three different breakfasts.[6] One was instant oatmeal with milk and sugar. Another was traditional, unprocessed steel-cut oats—the sort your grandmother would recognize. The third breakfast was an omelet.

The worst breakfast was the instant oats. After eating it, the boys' blood sugar and insulin levels soared, followed a couple of hours later by a crash as blood sugar levels fell below where they had started. This crash was accompanied by a surge of the stress hormone adrenaline. The boys felt tired, hungry, and irritable. At lunch they each ate a whopping 620 calories more than those who had had the omelet.

From personal experience I know how this feels. If I eat toast or cereal, I get hungry by midmorning. But if I eat, say, scrambled eggs for breakfast (even if it's the same number of calories), they keep me going well into the afternoon.

In another study, Ludwig put twenty-one overweight young men on diets ranging from low-fat to low-carb.[7] Despite eating exactly the same number of calories, those on the low-carb diet burned 325 calories more per day than those on the low-fat diet. This is about as much energy as you would burn in forty minutes of jogging.

"By the Time You Are Fifty, You Are Going to Have the Body You Deserve"

This is what Bob Smietana used to eat:

Breakfast: cereal, muffins, coffee (several cups)
Lunch: hamburger, pizza, french fries, soda
Dinner (on the way home in the car): two double cheese-
    burgers, big fries, soda

This fatty, carb-driven diet is typical of what many people eat on a regular basis. It's not as though we don't know those big bags of chocolate are supposed to be for sharing, or that that blueberry muffin won't count as one of our five daily servings of fruits and vegetables. It's just that this kind of stuff is so much easier to eat . . . even if it does leave us feeling bloated one second and starving the next.

Smietana is a journalist based in Chicago. He is an articulate, self-deprecating, middle-class kind of guy, with two teenage children, a happy marriage, and a successful career. During the time when he was on calorie overload, he had a lot on his plate, meta-phorically speaking—his work was stressful, and he was worried about his wife, who had been ill. Carb-filled, convenient fast food was a comfort.

Except it wasn't, because he was bad-tempered all the time, which wasn't like him. "I called myself 'Angry Bob,' " he says, look-ing back. "I was irritated constantly. Frustrated. Little things would set me off. My tension level had grown over time." He wasn't sleep-ing well, he says, and "I was making mistakes at work. My thinking wasn't clear." Sleep problems and mental fuzziness are both symp-toms of blood sugar issues, but most people don't make the con-nection.

He was in his midforties. He weighed over 280 pounds (he doesn't know for sure, because after that point he refused to get on the scale). And he didn't like what he could see in the mirror. Not long after this, he was diagnosed with type 2 diabetes.

"The minute the diagnosis came, it was terrifying," recalls Smie-tana. He describes it now as a teachable moment. "I wanted to live to see my daughter get married. I wanted to be around to enjoy my grandchildren. But I knew I was walking slowly toward an early death.

"Changing your diet and your habits is such a huge thing," he says. "You think, 'I can't do that.' You can't get started because you think it is too hard. The mountain is too big."

How did he do it? "Bit by bit. By moving in that direction and not thinking too much about how big this was. But it started with my own fear. The fear was a strength."

The first thing he did was get rid of the unhealthful carbohy-drates. The second thing he did was eat more vegetables. His calorie intake plummeted. "The more I did it, the less I liked the wrong things." He lost 90 pounds.

The man who used to be a regular at his local McDonald's drive-through took up walking. "I will go for a walk now. Even if the world is on fire, I will go for a walk, because I know that is what I need to do." His next goal is to run a marathon.

"I am a great believer in habit," says Smietana. "Once you do something over and over again, it becomes automatic and you stop thinking about it." He eats at the same time every day, he eats the same things, and he walks at the same time every day.

Looking back at how he used to live, he thinks we've become disconnected from our bodies. "We are on the phone or living virtual lives. We don't think about the physical side of life. We don't understand how our bodies work. Most people don't know what their pancreas does. What insulin is." Now he can tell when his blood sugar is going out of balance. "I can tell immediately if I haven't exercised. My emotions are heightened—be it excitement or anger or angst."

It's easy to like Smietana. He is a thoughtful guy who quietly and with determination dieted and walked his way back to health. He makes a vivid comparison with that other American obsession, the automobile. "In my twenties I had a car and I knew how to fix it—how to change a tire, for instance. Now I have no connection to it at all—we just replace our cars when something goes wrong. We expect to be able to do the same with our bodies, but we can't."

In 2015 his doctor—who was supportive throughout his diet—took him off his diabetes medication. And "Angry Bob" has disappeared.

Blood Sugar: The Toxic Time Bomb

Although being obese can lead to type 2 diabetes, as it did with Bob, it's not inevitable. You can be overweight without being diabetic. You can also be diabetic without being overweight. In fact, being a skinny type 2 diabetic can be more dangerous than being a fat one. The real problem, as we'll see, is not how much fat you carry but where it gets deposited. If you lay down fat in the wrong places, it can lead to high blood sugar, with all its potential complications, including the loss of a limb.

When I was a medical student I used to assist at operations. I say "assist," but all I really did was hold a retractor and laugh at the surgeon's jokes. I've watched plenty of successes and failures play out inside the operating room. But one of the saddest and most gruesome operations I attended was the removal of a patient's foot.

The patient was a man in his early fifties called Richard. I went to see him before his operation to take a medical history. I found him lying in bed with his two feet sticking out from under the sheets, "because I want to enjoy them for as long as I can." Richard, a successful lawyer, was frightened but trying not to show it. He was a loving husband and a proud father. A couple of years earlier he'd found himself becoming increasingly tired and lethargic. He went to see his doctor, had tests done, and discovered he was a type 2 diabetic.

Richard started taking pills, but soon progressed to insulin injections. He received no dietary advice, apart from being told to eat low-fat food and fill his plate with plenty of potatoes and pasta. He put on more and more weight.

Then one day he banged the side of his foot against a chair. He developed a little blister. This got bigger. Then it got infected. It was downhill from there. "It was all so quick," I remember him saying. "I had no idea that it would get so bad so fast."

His surgeon attempted to repair what was now a gaping ulcer on his foot with a skin graft taken from elsewhere on his body, but it failed. Richard was advised that he would have to have his foot removed.

He told me he was in shock when he heard the news. Terrified, he didn't know what to say. He went home and told his wife. She broke down and cried.

A day after first meeting Richard I went to the operating room and watched the surgeon remove his foot, which was then carried away to be disposed of. He spent months in the hospital recovering, and I never saw him again.

What Raised Blood Sugar Does to Your Body

Your Blood Vessels

The problem for Richard was that the high levels of sugar in his blood had stuck to proteins in the walls of his blood vessels, making them stiffer and less flexible. This, in time, had led to the buildup of scar tissue—plaque—inside his blood vessels. It had also damaged his nerves, so he could no longer feel pain when he bashed his foot.

If you'd looked inside Richard's eyes or the arteries supplying blood to his heart, you would have seen further damage. Diabetes is a major cause of blindness and more than doubles your risk of having a heart attack or stroke. It is also a leading cause of impotence in men.

And you don't have to have blood sugars in the diabetic range for damage to occur. In a big Australian study that followed more than ten thousand men and women for a number of years, researchers found that although being diabetic more than doubled the risk of dying, simply having blood sugar levels in the "impaired fasting glucose" range increased the risk of premature death by over 60 percent.[8]

Your Brain

My father started becoming confused toward the end of his life. He found it increasingly hard to remember names and was constantly forgetting conversations we'd had only a few hours before. He was convinced he was rich (which he wasn't) and began to give away money to strangers with hard-luck stories whom he met in bars and restaurants. I suspect he was showing early signs of dementia, which may well have been linked to his diabetes.

We've known for many years that diabetics have an increased risk of dementia (partly because of blood supply problems), but it's only recently that we've seen just how big the risk really is. In a recent study in Japan that followed more than one thousand men and women for fifteen years, researchers found that being diabetic doubled the risk of dementia.[9]

Dr. Suzanne de La Monte, a neuropathologist at Brown University, says that diabetes doesn't inevitably lead to dementia, but it's certainly an important factor. "Alzheimer's disease occurs in people without diabetes, and vice versa," she says. "But I think type 2 diabetes is pushing up rates of Alzheimer's disease like crazy."

Your Looks

Last and by no means least, raised blood sugar will make you look older by attacking the collagen and elastin molecules in your skin; this in turn makes your face saggy and wrinkled.

In a striking demonstration of this, researchers from Leiden University in the Netherlands measured the blood sugar of more than six hundred volunteers.[10] They then asked a group of independent assessors to try to guess their age. People with low blood sugar were scored as looking significantly younger than their real age, while those with high blood sugar were assessed as looking significantly older. The researchers estimate that every additional one-point increase in blood sugar adds five months to your perceived age.

Diabetes—The Physical Costs

★ Hypertension: 70 percent of diabetics also require medication for blood pressure.

★ Cholesterol: 65 percent of diabetics require medication to reduce their cholesterol.

★ Heart attacks: Diabetics, even when on medication, are twice as likely to be hospitalized, be crippled, or die from a heart attack.

★ Stroke: Diabetics are one and a half times more likely to suffer a debilitating stroke.

★ Blindness and eye problems: Diabetes is the number one cause of preventable blindness in the developed world.

★ Impotence: Diabetes is also the number one cause of impotence.

★ Dementia: Having diabetes doubles the risk of dementia.

★ Kidney disease: Diabetes is the cause in half of all new cases of kidney failure; most people on dialysis are diabetics.

★ Amputations: If you exclude trauma (such as from car accidents), diabetes is the commonest cause of limb amputations in the United States. Rates of diabetes-related amputations are soaring in countries such as Vietnam and India.

CHAPTER TWO

How Do You Solve a Problem Like Diabetes?

S O IF YOU'VE GOT TYPE 2 DIABETES OR PREDIABETES, can you reverse it?

This is a question that Roy Taylor answers with an emphatic yes. He is professor of medicine and metabolism at Newcastle University, where he also runs the Diabetes Research Group. He is slim and active, and with a dry sense of humor.

While his supporters say his very low-calorie diet has turned their lives around, he's met a lot of opposition. The first time he tried to publish a paper about his findings, it was turned down—the journal editors didn't believe the results.

"People don't think it is real," says Dr. Taylor. "Or they think that yes, you might be able to do it in a freak study, but it is not relevant. What you were told as a medical student and what you have been told your entire medical career is that people with type 2 diabetes get steadily worse and eventually end up on insulin. There are plenty of articles in the medical press that state firmly that the first thing someone ought to do when they are told they have type 2 is accept the diagnosis. And then I come along and tell them that might not be true."

Recently one of his high-profile critics approached him after a lecture. "I was wrong," he told Dr. Taylor. "You were right." If Dr. Taylor were the type to punch the air, he might have done so.

What makes resistance to Dr. Taylor's research so surprising is that for many years there has been clear evidence that type 2 diabetes can be reversed through dramatic weight loss—most notably through bariatric (weight loss) surgery.

Dr. Taylor came across the link between bariatric surgery and diabetes in the 1980s when he visited Greenville, North Carolina, a city with very high rates of obesity. One of the medical professionals he met there was a surgeon named Walter Pories. He not only did weight loss surgery on obese patients but also conducted long-term follow-up studies to find out what happened to them afterward. One study followed 608 seriously obese patients for fourteen years.[11] Not everyone improved, but in most cases the weight loss was spectacular. By the end of the first year the patients had, on average, lost a third of their total body weight (100 pounds), a weight loss that they maintained till the end of the study, fourteen years later.

Along with the drop in weight were a significant decline in blood pressure, improvements in sleep, and a big drop in the risk of dying from heart disease. Perhaps the most impressive change, however, was seen in those who had blood sugar problems. Of the 608 patients in the study, 161 had type 2 diabetes and 150 had impaired glucose tolerance (prediabetes). For most of these patients there was an immediate and dramatic fall in blood sugar levels soon after surgery. As the researchers observed, "The diabetes cleared rapidly, generally in a matter of days, to the degree that most diabetic bariatric surgical patients were discharged without any anti-diabetic medications."

One patient, who previously had been on huge doses of insulin, was able to stop her insulin within a week of surgery, and within three months her blood sugars had returned to normal. Even more impressive, fourteen years later she, like 83 percent of the former diabetics, still had normal blood sugar levels.

The patients who didn't respond as well were those who had been diabetic for many years before the surgery. But those who were prediabetic—with blood sugar high but not yet in the danger zone—had the best results of all. In 99 percent of them, blood sugar levels went back to normal and stayed there.

Weight loss surgery, it ought to be said, is not an easy option. Although death rates are low, patients sometimes have to be readmitted to the hospital to treat infections or because their incisions don't heal properly. The operation can also lead to "dumping syndrome" after eating, which is as unpleasant as it sounds: heart rate soars, there's a feeling of butterflies in the stomach, and profound diarrhea occurs.

The researchers had noticed that after surgery patients had changes in gut hormones, the chemicals our bodies produce that control appetite. So they assumed that the surgery itself had somehow changed the hormones, and that this was why the patients' blood sugar levels dropped. Dr. Taylor, however, was not convinced. "I know about gut hormones—they are very important, but they have limited effect on metabolic changes. I knew right away this claim had to be wrong. But it became the established belief, the belief throughout the scientific world: a change in gut hormones explains why blood sugars return to normal after surgery."

He thought there was a completely different explanation—one that could explain why many overweight people don't get diabetes, while many slim people do.

The Worst Places to Pile on the Fat: It's Not Where You Think

Insulin decides *whether* you get fat, but it is an enzyme called lipoprotein lipase, LPL, that decides *where* you get fat.

We don't become fat all over—we don't have fat foreheads, for example—but rather we accumulate fat in certain places. And whether fat will accumulate around your middle, your thighs, your bottom, or your hips depends largely on LPL. Once activated, this enzyme will, with the help of insulin, suck the fat out of your blood and stick it in storage.

Men tend to have more LPL in the fat cells of their bellies, which is why they tend to put on fat around their waists.

Women, on the other hand, are more likely to have active LPL in the fat cells of the hips and the bottom, which is why the fat piles on there.

The good news is that LPL is also found in muscles. If you activate the LPL in your muscles by exercising, then any surplus calories you take in are more likely to be dumped there and burned as energy, instead of stored as fat.

A few years ago, while making a documentary called *The Truth About Exercise*, I took part in an experiment at Glasgow University in Scotland to demonstrate the difference even a modest amount of exercise can make.

The experiment consisted of eating a large, greasy breakfast full of fried foods, including bacon, eggs, and the Scottish specialty haggis. An hour later I had some blood taken by Dr. Jason Gill. He then put my blood into a sophisticated centrifuge and spun it down to separate the red cells from the plasma. When this was done he showed me, floating on top of my plasma, a murky layer of fat. This was the fat that I had eaten at breakfast and which was now traveling around my arteries. He then asked me to go for a brisk one-hour walk, which I did.

The following morning I did exactly the same thing as I had done the day before: I ate a greasy breakfast, after which my blood was taken and spun down. This time, however, the layer of fat on top of my plasma was much thinner. The walk the previous afternoon had switched on genes in my leg muscles that activated the LPL enzymes in those muscles, which in turn sucked much of the fat out of my blood.

Unfortunately, most of us don't go for long, vigorous

walks after a meal, or indeed at any other time. A far more likely fate for the calories from a big meal is that the insulin in your blood will direct them into fat cells. Some will become subcutaneous fat, the fat that gathers just under the skin on your bottom, thighs, and arms. That is relatively harmless. But the rest will become visceral fat, which is a hidden fat that wraps itself around your heart, liver, and digestive system. Because this fat lies inside the body, rather than on the surface where you can see it, you can appear to be relatively slim. People with such an accumulation of visceral fat are known as TOFIs—thin on the outside, fat on the inside. I used to be one of them.

Fatty Liver and Pancreas—
The Heart of the Problem

Visceral fat is particularly dangerous because it invades organs such as your liver and pancreas. We don't think of our livers as being "fatty," but the liver is actually one of the first places that fat gets stored. It is like a checking account at the bank: a quick and easy place to put away spare cash. But it is an account with, as Dr. Taylor puts it, punishingly high fees, because it can lead to all sorts of problems—not just abnormal blood sugar levels but also nonalcoholic fatty liver disease (NAFLD). Thirty percent of Europeans and Americans have NAFLD, which can lead to cirrhosis and liver failure. It is the commonest cause of liver disease in the West.

Dr. Taylor's research suggests that it is the buildup of

fat inside the liver and pancreas that causes all the trouble. These two organs are responsible for controlling our insulin and blood sugar levels. As they get clogged up with fat they stop communicating with each other. Eventually your body stops producing insulin and you become a type 2 diabetic.

Dr. Taylor also argues that we have our own "personal fat threshold," which can be thought of as a tipping point that decides how much fat you can accumulate before it starts to overflow into your liver and pancreas.[12] In some people this threshold seems to be set high, while in others it's surprisingly low; genetics appears to play some role in what any individual's threshold is.

The good news is that whatever your personal fat threshold may be, if you drain the fat out of your liver and pancreas (and the diet in this book does just that), then you can reverse your diabetes and restore your blood sugar level to normal. The bad news is that if you *don't* do this, then you will not only get the complications of diabetes but may also permanently damage your liver.

"People Would Tell Me, 'Lorna, You Have Nothing to Worry About—You're Thin' "

Lorna Norman's doctor was shocked when a blood test revealed that Lorna had blood sugar problems. Lorna is a vegetarian and had always eaten healthfully. She walked her dogs every day. She swam regularly. She had never had a health scare before. Apart from tiredness—which was what had prompted her to go to her doctor in the first place—she had no symptoms.

After seeing the doctor, she was sent to a nurse who told her not to worry and to keep on doing what she'd been doing. "In hindsight," says Lorna, "that was the last thing I needed to do." And that was common mistake number one.

"People would tell me, 'Lorna, you have nothing to worry about. You're thin. You look fine.' " That's common mistake number two.

She continued eating plenty of carbohydrates—pasta, bread, baked potatoes. That was common mistake number three. "Now I know that was completely the wrong thing to eat, but that was what the experts were telling me to do," she acknowledges.

For several years her blood sugar levels hovered around the borderline mark. But then they gradually began to creep up. At that point she weighed 133 pounds. At five foot four, this isn't overweight. But—and this is key—her excess weight had a tendency to sit around her middle.

On her next visit to the doctor she got the news she had been dreading: she was diabetic. Her doctor told her she needed to immediately start on medication. That was common mistake number four.

When Lorna told her doctor about Roy Taylor's research suggesting that very low-calorie dieting could take her blood sugar levels back down to normal, he was skeptical. "He told me, 'You are not overweight and your body mass index is fine' "—it was a little under 23, which is within the normal range. " 'You really shouldn't be on this kind of diet,' he told me. He thought it was nonsense"—common mistake number five.

She decided to go ahead with the very low-calorie diet nonetheless. "I just thought, 'I am going to have a stab at anything that stops me from going on medication.' " She pauses, then adds with a laugh, "My daughter might say I am a control freak."

After four weeks her body mass index, or BMI, had dropped to 19. She made sure she was getting enough of the right nutrients, and she drank three quarts of water a day. It wasn't all smooth sailing, however—frequent tests showed that her blood sugar levels improved initially, but then started going up again. "I thought I must be one of those people for whom it didn't work," she recalls. But that was common mistake number six.

She continued with the plan—and she stopped having her blood sugar levels tested so often, which helped her to stop worrying. She also took up yoga and meditation ("I would put the laundry in and meditate until the end-of-cycle signal sounded"). Her stress levels fell, which also brought down her levels of the stress hormone cortisol, which increases blood sugar.

Amazingly, she managed to do all this and still cater to three other adults in the house. She even continued to do all the cooking. "I would do their meals and then sit down to whatever little plate of food that I was having."

At her lightest, she was 119 pounds. "Lots of people commented on how thin I looked, but frankly I didn't care. People are more likely to say something about how you look than they are to congratulate you for not having a life-threatening illness any longer. It's very peculiar."

By the end of two months she was diabetes-free. The crucial factor was probably that her waist measurement had reduced from 34 inches to 30 inches—a sign that her stores of visceral fat had decreased significantly.

What's Wrong With Just Taking Pills?

As we all know, losing weight and keeping it off requires effort. So if your doctor tells you, "Yes, you have type 2 diabetes, but it's easily treatable with pills," then you are probably going to take the easy way out.

But diabetes is rarely that simple. Even when the condition is treated with medication, being a diabetic can take ten years off your life.

It will also cost you, or whoever has to cover your medical expenses, a great deal of money. It's not just the cost of the drugs, the cost of treating the complications, and the time off work. Having a diagnosis of type 2 diabetes will also make getting life insurance harder and more expensive. Even travel insurance may cost more because of the increased risks. In the United States it's estimated that type 2 diabetes costs the country at least $245 billion each year.

The bestselling anti-diabetes drug on the market at the moment is metformin, with sales of nearly $2 billion a year. It has been around for so long and used on so many people that you would imagine it must be really effective. Yet a recent meta-analysis that looked at the results of thirteen randomized controlled trials involving more than thirteen thousand patients could find little compelling evidence that taking the drug reduces heart attacks, decreases the likelihood of leg amputation, or improves life expectancy.[13]

At least metformin can lead to modest weight reduction (possibly because common side effects include nausea), but it is normally only the first step on a road that leads to more powerful and expensive anti-diabetes drugs. And most of these other drugs, including insulin, promote hunger, which makes patients fatter. As one expert told me, "The more aggressively we treat them, the fatter they get."

The current situation with diabetes reminds me, in some ways, of the first television documentary I ever made, back in the early 1990s. It was called *Ulcer Wars*, and it was about a young Australian doctor called Barry Marshall. At that time stomach ulcers were a very common and painful condition caused, as everyone knew, by the production of too much acid in the stomach. It was widely believed that the increased acid was the result of stress and a poor lifestyle. You had brought this condition on yourself by living badly.

Fortunately, the wonderful pharmaceutical companies had developed drugs that could reduce the symptoms by reducing the acid levels in your stomach. But because this was an incurable disease, you had to go on taking expensive drugs for the rest of your life or the ulcers would return.

Dr. Marshall, however, was not convinced by this explanation. He believed that stomach ulcers were actually caused by a previously unknown bacterium, *Helicobacter pylori*, which he and a colleague, Robin Warren, had discovered in the stomachs they had had to remove from unfortunate patients whose ulcers had burst.

They tried, and failed, to infect animals in the lab with *H. pylori*, so in the end Marshall decided to infect himself. He didn't tell his wife because, as he candidly told me, "she would have tried to stop me."

Before doing anything he persuaded a colleague to push an endoscopic tube down his throat and take a good look at his stomach. It was completely normal. Then he asked a technician to brew up a beaker of bacteria (grown from an infected patient's stomach) and swallowed it in one shot—it was hardly the sort of thing you would want to sip. A few days later he became ill and vomited. He was thrilled.

He had himself endoscoped again, and this time the surgeon saw patches of inflammation. He took samples of Marshall's stomach, and when they looked at the samples through a microscope, they saw bacteria swarming through the tissue. Marshall's wife insisted that he stop the experiment, so he took a cocktail of antibiotics and Pepto-Bismol (which is mildly toxic to bacteria); a few days later his symptoms improved.

By the time I made my documentary, Barry Marshall and others had treated a lot of patients and shown not only that most stomach ulcers could be cured with antibiotics but also that doing so would reduce patients' chance of developing stomach cancer. Yet few doctors were listening and the only response to my film from the medical profession was a review in the *British Medical Journal* that described it as "one-sided and tendentious"—medical-speak for "garbage." Within a few years, however, the evidence was so overwhelming and patient demand so great that use of antibiotic therapy for ulcers became widespread. In 2000 Barry Marshall and Robin Warren won the Nobel Prize for Medicine.

As with stomach ulcers, you can certainly control diabetes with drugs. But wouldn't it be far better to treat the underlying cause? If you had an infection, wouldn't you want to get rid of it before it progresses, rather than merely treat the symptoms?

"Doctors Will Argue That They're Too Busy to Monitor Weight Loss. But It Could Save Them a Hell of a Lot of Time in the Long Term if They Did"

It took Colin Beattie four months to wear down his doctor. Luckily, he is a politician—he's a member of the Scottish Parliament—so he knows how to make an argument. And repeat it. Again and again.

The sixty-three-year-old had been diagnosed with type 2 diabetes four years before, and at the beginning he barely gave the diagnosis a second thought. He was told to take one tablet of metformin in the morning and one in the evening. Two years later—because his blood sugar levels were still rising—his dose needed to be doubled. So now he was on four tablets a day. The next thing he knew, he was being put on statins. Toward the end of 2013, on his next visit to the doctor, he was informed that his blood pressure was too high, and another pill was prescribed, this time to dilate the vessels supplying blood to his kidneys.

It was at this point that Colin began to seriously wonder about the ever-mounting pile of pills. "I started thinking, 'Hang on. Is this what life is going to be like? More and more tablets?' "

Colin did some research. He discovered Dr. Taylor's work on very low-calorie diets and the potential to reverse type 2 diabetes. His doctor wasn't thrilled about the idea. "He was clearly worried he would have a flood of people coming into the office asking for help on the diet and that his office wouldn't be able to cope," he says.

Until then, the dietary advice Colin had been given was basic: eat more fruit and vegetables, avoid fatty food. "It seemed," says Colin, "like an ordinary well-intentioned admonition to eat better." Predictably, Colin pretty much ignored the advice (well, you would, wouldn't you, if your doctor seems to think you should keep on taking the pills and not worry?). "I tended to eat what I could, when I could," he says. "Fish and chips, steak pie, snacks between meals . . . a typical Scotsman's diet," he says.

Gradually his doctor tired of the former investment banker sitting opposite him brandishing bundles of facts and figures about why a very low-calorie diet could work. Reluctantly he gave Colin the go-ahead and agreed to monitor his progress.

What Colin did—and I think this was key to his success—was to approach the diet as though it were a pharmaceutical regime. This was *prescription weight loss.* Because his day-to-day life is so high-pressured and variable, he decided to use prepackaged diet meals, as opposed to eating real food. A typical day was oatmeal for breakfast, soup for lunch, and a diet bar plus a plate of steamed vegetables for dinner. That added up to 800 calories.

"I did two things that I think helped," he says now. "I made sure everyone knew I was going to do it—including the press. That helped keep the pressure on me. And I was absolutely determined that I wasn't going to break the diet. I knew that if I did, it would be easier to break it the next time and the next time. I absolutely stuck to it until the last day." (After that last day, he went out and ate a steak pie. The less said about that the better, but it goes to show he's human.)

Over eight weeks he lost 44 pounds. His waist shrank from 40 inches to 34 inches. By the end he was free of his medication. And, despite the occasional steak pie, Colin has managed to keep the weight off. When it creeps up a pound or two he cuts back. He is on a mission now to spread the word about low-calorie diets. He has been amazed by how many people have told him that they, too, have type 2 diabetes and are shocked by how little support they get.

There are 236,000 type 2 diabetics in Scotland (not counting the people who don't know they've got it). Among those newly diagnosed last year were five children under four years old. "Doctors will argue that they are busy and don't have the time to monitor weight loss. But it could save them a hell of a lot of time in the long term if they did deal with it," Colin points out.

The Newcastle Study

Dr. Taylor was pretty sure that if he could get a diabetic patient to lose enough weight, this would drain the fat out of the pancreas and liver and reverse the diabetes. But because so many other doctors were skeptical, he knew he was going to have to put together a very convincing case.

First he needed to be able to measure what was actually happening to the levels of liver and pancreatic fat in his patients. Kieran Hollingsworth, a physicist in his department, had already adapted an MRI machine to measure liver fat. When Dr. Taylor asked him whether it could be done for the pancreas as well, Hollingsworth stared up at the ceiling and thought for a moment before saying, "Yes."

Next Dr. Taylor needed money to do a trial. "I was very

fortunate," he said, "to get money from the nonprofit Diabetes UK. They thought it was extremely unlikely to work, but one particular person there thought it sounded interesting and managed to persuade the rest of the committee. It wasn't much—enough for a small one-year study."

With the funding in place they recruited fourteen patients.[14] Three of the volunteers dropped out early for a variety of reasons. The remaining eleven were taken off their normal diabetes drugs and put on a strict regime of 800 calories a day, which consisted of liquid diet drinks and nonstarchy vegetables.

In the first week they lost an average of 8 pounds, and most reported finding the diet surprisingly easy. "Much to my astonishment, the hunger seems to disappear in forty-eight hours," Dr. Taylor told me.

As the fat clogging up their livers melted away, their symptoms improved. "The liver seemed to be fine after seven days and got better as time went by. The pancreas was slower to respond. It was a little better after seven days and then steadily improved over the next eight weeks—and that was the magic thing."

The volunteers stuck to the 800-calorie regime, and in just eight weeks—a remarkably short time—lost an average of 33 pounds. They also lost nearly 5 inches from their waist. By the end their blood sugar levels were all back in the nondiabetic range.

Dr. Taylor was astonished. "It was electrifying. Amazingly more definitive that I ever dreamed it would be."

Alan's Story

Alan, fifty-six and married with four sons, was part of that study. He weighed 213 pounds when he was diagnosed with diabetes and essentially told, "You've got it, deal with it." When he heard that Dr. Taylor was looking for volunteers, he leaped at the chance. His own doctor was less enthusiastic, telling him, "Don't feel bad when you fail."

But Alan didn't fail. "I never felt that I was flagging or wanted to give up. I felt like a pioneer, that what I was doing was important."

In eight weeks Alan lost 29 pounds, almost 14 percent of his starting weight. Three years later, he has kept most of that weight off and his blood sugar measurements remain in the healthy range.

"I'm no angel. I still have take-out food, wine, cheese, beer. I have a special black shirt that used to fit like a second skin. I put it on every so often to see if it still fits. As long as it fits, I'm doing fine."

Alan, like the other volunteers in this first study, had been recently diagnosed with type 2 diabetes. Would it work with people who had been diabetic for longer? In a follow-up study published in 2015, Dr. Taylor's team tested the diet on twenty-nine people with type 2 diabetes, some of whom had been diabetic for more than eight years and some who had been diabetic for more than four years but less than eight years.[15] Again they found that people were surprisingly good at sticking to the diet and got great results. In this trial 87 percent of the group who had been diabetic for between four and eight years and 50 percent of the group who had been diabetic for more than eight years managed to get their fasting blood sugars back to normal without medication.

So does Dr. Taylor have any concerns about people doing a very low-calorie weight loss program outside a clinical setting?

"None," he replied, "except for two specific reservations, both of those related to drugs. If you are on antihypertensive medication, for high blood pressure, then you should discuss with your doctors either cutting down or stopping the medication before you start dieting. Your blood pressure is going to drop, and it could go too low if the drugs are continued. Similarly, there are some glucose-lowering drugs, ones that begin with the letter G, such as glyburide and gliclazide, which may have to be stopped because in conjunction with the diet they can push your blood glucose abnormally low."

What would he say to those who worry about the potential dangers of going on a very low-calorie diet for two months? "The anxieties about fasting have been grossly exaggerated, and it partly relates to poor-quality 400-calorie diets that were used long ago in the U.S. for very long periods of time," he notes. "With a balanced 800 calories for eight weeks I have absolutely no qualms at all, though ideally people should discuss their plans with their doctor or diabetes team to get personal medical advice."

So what does he think about doing it with real food rather

than diet shakes or bars? "I'd rather people did. When the diet was first talked about publicly, seventy-seven individuals did it on their own initiative, and half of them did it by eating real food. They lost the same amount of weight as we had achieved under controlled conditions in our studies. It can be done."

Dr. Taylor's team has shown that it is possible to reverse type 2 diabetes in motivated people. The really important thing now is to test this idea on a larger scale, find out who it's most suitable for, and, crucially, see what happens in the long term. He and colleagues including Mike Lean, professor of human nutrition at Glasgow University, are currently involved in a much bigger study. Patients volunteering for DiReCT (Diabetes Remission Clinical Trial) are randomly assigned to either the best currently available type 2 diabetes care or the 800-calorie-a-day diet. The trial will run for five years and involve more than thirty doctors' practices across the United Kingdom.

In the meantime, many individuals have been taking matters into their own hands.

"I Was Ready to Die, and Suddenly I Hear About a Cure for This Disease!"

Carlos Cervantes should be dead. There is no question in his mind about it. Indeed, just before the fifty-five-year-old discovered Dr. Taylor's work—totally by chance; I'll tell you how in a second—he had concluded that his time was up. "I had decided that this was a good summer to die," he tells me. "It wasn't a low point. It was a realistic assessment of my situation."

This is what Carlos was up against: at his heaviest he weighed 300 pounds, his waist measured 56 inches, his toes were beginning to turn black, he had a fungal infection in his ear, and his doctor had warned him that an out-of-control foot ulcer meant he was looking at amputation. There were crutches beside the bed in his remote house on the slopes of Mount St. Helens in Washington State. Insulin injections were no longer working. When he tested his blood sugar, the machine could not process the reading—it turned out to be because the number was so high it was off the scale.

There are lots of reasons why this soft-spoken man was in a fog of despair. Here are a few of them:

His doctor had given up on him.

"It was very traumatic," he recalls. "I wasn't getting any help and I didn't know what was wrong with me. I was as sick as sick can be." Carlos, who has a dark sense of humor, had nicknamed metformin "MakeFatMan" because for him a side effect was even more weight gain.

He had raging type 2 diabetes.

When fungus starts living off the sugar in your blood, you're not talking borderline symptoms anymore. According to every medical professional he spoke to, type 2 diabetes is a progressive illness, and he seemed to be in the final stages.

He had done lots of diets in the past, and none of them had worked.

Following the death of his mother from cancer when he was five, Carlos used food to compensate for the emotional loss. He was nine when, overweight and miserable, he began his first attempt at weight loss—the Atkins Diet. "That didn't work for me," he laughs now. "Nothing ever really worked. I would lose weight and then it would all come back." He had a weakness for chocolate brownies, and then some.

He was depressed and stressed. He was squeezed emotionally dry by major bereavements, a promising real estate business had been devastated by the credit crunch, and he was beset by financial worries.

And then one day he heard about Dr. Taylor's diet in a two-minute news item on the Al Jazeera cable channel. "I was ready to die, and suddenly I hear about a cure for this disease!" What was that like? "I think I busted a hole in the roof!" he replies. "I couldn't believe what I had heard." Carlos began doing his own research online and found an email address for Dr. Taylor. He says, "I knew my doctor would tell me that it would not work. I decided to take matters into my own hands."

Carlos couldn't bear the diet shakes that were recommended, so mostly he ate real food—just different kinds and a lot less of it, including vegetables, fruit, lean chicken, and salad. Everything was carefully weighed out every day—if he had cheese, he would measure out a sliver. On the tenth day his blood sugar dropped for the first time. After sixty-four days he had lost 67 pounds, the equivalent of an adult Irish setter dog. His target was 173 pounds, and by the time he reached it, his diabetes had disappeared. "It cured me beyond my expectations," he says. "I would even call it a superhuman cure."

Since then he has changed the way he eats—mostly. He estimates he eats 95 percent healthful food and 5 percent junk. "At the center of my plate is a pile of steamed fresh vegetables, and around that is healthful grains. On the side is a piece of fish or chicken." He still occasionally eats chocolate cake or ice cream or tortilla chips, but he says it does not affect him in the way it used to. "As a diabetic, I couldn't eat any of those things. The diet cleaned out my liver and pancreas. It's not so easy for me to gain weight anymore. I can get real skinny quickly. It's as though my body is working metabolically like a young man's again."

He's now wearing pants with a 32-inch waist. "I like the person I see in the mirror now," he says. "Although sometimes it is hard to recognize myself. I was morbidly obese my entire adult life."

He is a diabetes buddy at a nearby support group for people with issues around food, and he says, "I will go to any lengths to bring the message of hope and recovery to any diabetic out there." Make no mistake about it—he is deadly serious.

CHAPTER THREE

Are You at Risk for Type 2 Diabetes?

HERE IS A CLOSE BUT NOT INEVITABLE LINK BE-tween weight and the risk of developing blood sugar problems. It also depends on your age, gender, and ethnicity.

If you are of white European descent, you are more than twice as likely to develop type 2 diabetes if you have a BMI over 30 than if your BMI is less than 25.

Men, because they have a greater tendency to put on weight around the abdominal area, are more likely to develop type 2 diabetes at a lower BMI.

If you are of South Asian, Chinese, Afro-Caribbean, or black African descent, then you are at increased risk. You are likely to get diabetes at a lower BMI earlier in life, and to go from being prediabetic to diabetic twice as quickly. This is one reason why in countries such as Vietnam, which have

Are You at Risk for Type 2 Diabetes?

1. Do you have a diabetic parent, brother, or sister?   **1 point**

2. Are you being treated for hypertension?   **1 point**

3. Are you from a nonwhite ethnic background?   **1 point**

4. Are you aged 50 to 59?   **1 point**

5. Are you over 60?   **2 points**

6. Is your waist over 35 but less than 42 inches?   **1 point**

7. Is your waist over 42 inches?   **2 points**

8. Is your Body Mass Index (BMI) 31-35?   **1 point**

9. Is your BMI over 35?   **2 points**

Measure your waist around the belly button, not your trouser size.

To get your BMI score go to our website thebloodsugardiet .com, which will calculate it for you.

Add up your total score:

Less than 3 points: You have a low risk of becoming type 2 diabetic in the next 10 years.

3-5 points: You have a moderate risk of becoming diabetic and as you get older this risk will increase. Check your blood sugars and consider making lifestyle changes so you can reduce your risk.

Over 5 points: You are at high risk of becoming diabetic. You should definitely have your blood sugars tested and aim for lifestyle changes, such as significant weight loss and increased activity.

adopted a Western lifestyle, doctors are now amputating more limbs due to the complications of diabetes than they were because of injuries at the height of the Vietnam War.

A condition that used to occur mainly in older people is skewing younger. Type 2 diabetes is far more serious if you get it in your twenties or thirties than if you develop it later in life. As one expert told me, "A forty-five-year-old man who gets it is likely to have his first major complication just thirteen years later. People talk in terms of reduced life expectancy, but if you are a forty-five-year-old and you know that you might have to stop work early and be unable to support your family, that's scary."

"I Have Been Given Another Chance at Life"

Cassie was just twenty-four years old and pregnant when she was started on diabetes medication. She had developed what's called gestational diabetes when she was carrying her daughter, Grace.

Gestational diabetes is common; around 9 percent of pregnant women get it. No one knows why, but one theory is that hormones produced during pregnancy can block insulin receptors, making blood sugar levels rise. It normally disappears after the woman gives birth.

Cassie's blood sugar levels were so high that her doctor put her on insulin. She hoped things would get better after her daughter was born. But they didn't.

Like many people who have a complex relationship with food, Cassie is insightful about what happened next. "I got into this cycle of guilt—feeling guilty that I was a diabetic with a young child, guilty about what I ate. One fueled the other. In the end it seemed pointless to try to do anything about it—and then I ate more." She was training to be a nurse. At work she would see people with type 2 diabetes and all the complications that the illness brings, which just made her feel worse.

She was told to cut back on fatty foods, so she increased her consumption of carbs. Breakfast was pastries, cereal, toast. Lunch would be sandwiches. Dinner, more often than not, was take-out. She would eat in secret, as she was constantly hungry—perhaps because of all the insulin she was injecting. Over the next four years she put on a lot of weight.

When Cassie sent me an email, she was so desperate to change that she was considering weight loss surgery. She had tried every diet going, including Weight Watchers, and nothing had worked.

I wanted to help, but she was on such high doses of insulin that I was worried about what might happen. So I passed her details on to my wife, Clare, who's a general practitioner and sees a lot of diabetics.

Clare had a chat with Cassie and discovered that she had a supportive endocrinologist monitoring her condition. Also important was that she knew exactly how to adjust her insulin to avoid hypoglycemia (when the blood sugar drops dangerously low). Reassured, Clare gave Cassie the go-ahead. She explained the principles of the 800-calorie diet and discussed what foods Cassie could eat and those she couldn't. She offered regular email or phone support.

Cassie had no idea whether she would be able to stick to what sounded like a tough regime, but she had two powerful motivating forces. First was her daughter, Grace. She didn't want her little girl growing up with a mom who was ill and incapacitated. Second, she had hit rock bottom. "I had nothing to lose," she says.

What surprised her was that it didn't take long to get into a new habit. The first few days were tough—"It felt like my stomach was eating itself," she recalls—but she swiftly got into a routine that worked for her, with lots of protein and vegetables and no refined carbohydrates. In the evening she would eat a smaller portion of what her husband was eating—a stir-fry or a salad.

Amazingly, after just a week the hunger ended. For the first time in her life she was no longer obsessed with food. It was a revelation.

Within two weeks she was able to stop her insulin and metformin. She didn't need them because her blood sugars had returned to normal. And they've stayed that way ever since.

She remained on the diet for eight weeks and lost just over 44 pounds. "I feel amazing. I don't think about food anymore. I'm full of energy. Happy. I really do think I have been given another chance at life. I feel in control for the first time."

A couple of months after stopping her medications, she sent an email to say that after years of trying, she was pregnant again. "I had a conversation with my midwife, who said that some studies have shown that polycystic ovaries, which is what I have, can be caused by high amounts of insulin in the blood. She thinks that I got pregnant because I was able to come off my insulin. So I cannot thank you enough, because not only have you freed me from food and put me back in charge of my own life, but you have also helped me to make a little miracle possible—which I never thought would happen."

Stress: The Powerful Role It Plays

As Cassie clearly demonstrates, food is tied up with how we feel. Emotions such as stress, anger, fear, and anxiety make us reach for the cookie jar, which in turn will make our blood sugar go haywire.

Death of a loved one, divorce, work stress, unemployment—the more people I talked to for this book, the more I realized how much our emotions are linked to blood sugar. Almost everyone could date their problems back to emotional upheaval.

More than a century ago, Henry Maudsley, one of the founders of modern psychiatry, noted that blood sugar problems often followed sudden trauma. He reported the story of a soldier who, upon discovering that his wife was having an affair, immediately developed type 2 diabetes.[16] More recently, Walter Cannon, the scientist at Harvard who first came up with the term "fight-or-flight response," found that cats' blood sugar rose when they were frightened or stressed.[17]

So what is happening? Negative and stressful emotions, such as anger, frustration, or sadness, drive up levels of stress hormones in the body, including adrenaline and cortisol. These hormones are part of our fight-or-flight response, which evolved to help us survive in times of crisis by making glucose readily available to use as fuel. A study of nondiabetic bungee jumpers found that the stress of the jump caused blood sugar levels to rise significantly. This is just what you want if you're not diabetic. But if you have problems with blood sugar control, that's the opposite of what you want.

Stress-related hormones make muscles and tissues more insulin-resistant. They stimulate the liver to release more sugar into the blood, hinder the pancreas from making insulin, and block insulin's ability to get sugar into cells.

This whole scenario feeds frustration, sadness, and anger. To cheer yourself up, you eat more.

"The Father We Knew Had Disappeared in a Fog of Depression, Embarrassment, Lack of Confidence, and Pain"

Anthony and Ian Whitington didn't realize their father, Geoff, had fallen into a diabetes-related depression until it was almost too late. He had been diagnosed when he was fifty. "He just took it as yet another illness," recalls Anthony, "and so did we." They knew that he was on medication for high cholesterol and blood pressure. "But the diabetes news was a bit of a nonevent. It just seemed like more pills to take."

Geoff's doctor could have urged him to change his habits. But he didn't. He played it down. He told Geoff, who worked as a security guard on the night shift, that this was something he could live with, something he could manage. One reason doctors do this is that they know their dietary advice is likely to be ignored.

Busy doctors have developed a form of "learned helplessness." They know that standard dietary advice is rarely listened to or followed. They watch patients who don't change their eating habits pile on the weight, and then they have to prescribe more medication with a sense of resignation.

Geoff began a low-fat diet in a rather halfhearted way, but he didn't see much change and soon started eating in secret. Fast food may have been slowly killing him, but it was also his way of cheering himself up. He'd go to McDonald's and hide the wrappers before he got home, at which point he would sit down to an evening meal as though he had not eaten since lunchtime. His wife, Marion, who was trying to cook him healthier meals at home, had no idea that he was eating for two.

Eleven years after his diagnosis of type 2 diabetes he had an ulcer on his right foot and a collapsed arch on the left one. Both can lead to amputation. He had neuropathy in his fingers—he could touch hot things and not notice. He was becoming reclusive. "The father we knew had disappeared in a fog of depression, embarrassment, lack of confidence, and pain," says Anthony.

Anthony, who works in finance, and his brother, Ian, a documentary filmmaker, decided to stage an intervention. They came up with a plan to film their dad. They told him they were making a documentary about type 2 diabetes, but what they were really doing was trying to get him interested in life again. "Initially he just played along with it, thinking it was just another one of our crazy projects," laughs Anthony. The result was an incredibly moving—and funny—film called *Fixing Dad*.

Geoff is now diabetes-free. His readings used to be sky high. Now they are bouncing along in the normal range. How did Geoff do it? His sons put him on a very low-calorie diet and asked him to take a photograph on his phone of every meal (making him accountable for everything he ate). They weaned him off his traditional meals and introduced him to new ingredients. There were a lot of fights in the supermarket—"There was a lot of tension, a lot of arguments, because we are all stubborn," he admits—but he lost 18 pounds in the first two weeks.

Geoff's sons had researched the evidence on rapid weight loss and how it can reverse diabetes, and they believed that they could turn their father's blood sugar problems—and his depression—around. "We really clung to the idea that this was something potentially reversible. It was a real driving force. We told ourselves, 'It has fixed one person; maybe it can fix Dad too.' It was an important message—that this can be *reversed*."

Gradually exercise became part of Geoff's new life. He took up cycling. The exercise made him feel good about himself. As part of the film, his sons challenged him to try new physical activities—skydiving, white-water rafting.

In addition to losing 84 pounds, Geoff found that his mood gradually improved. "He is totally different now," says Anthony. "His aura, the way he projects himself—he has self-confidence. He believes he can do things." So much so that the man who spent the last decade mostly sitting at home now visits companies and tells their employees that they can change their health and their lives.

As noted above, Geoff had spent most of his career as a nighttime security guard. A study in 2010 tested nine healthy adults to see what effect sleep deprivation has on insulin resistance.[18] On one night, individuals were allowed to sleep for up to 8½ (the average was about 7 hours 34 minutes). On another night, they could sleep a maximum of 4 hours (with an average of 3 hours 46 minutes). The results show that in the sleep-deprived state there was evidence of insulin resistance: the internal production of sugar was higher, and clearance of glucose into muscle cells was lower.

Less than four hours is not much sleep. But then again, increased insulin resistance was seen in individuals after just one night of sleep deprivation. It's possible that less extreme sleep deprivation over long periods of time also poses hazards for the body.

Later on in the book I will give you some techniques to manage stress, which are likely to also help you sleep better.

CHAPTER FOUR

Going Low-Carb

I N CHAPTER ONE, I EXPLAINED WHY SO MANY EXPERTS now believe that the obsession with "low-fat everything" helped fuel an overconsumption of cheap and easily digestible carbohydrates, which in turn helped feed the recent surge in obesity.

Easily digestible carbohydrates include all forms of sugars (sugar-sweetened sodas make it particularly easy to consume huge amounts), many processed foods (sugars are now added to a huge number of them), as well as crackers, cakes, breakfast cereals, rice, pasta, and bread.

Despite this, the standard advice for type 2 diabetics continues to be, "Eat a low-fat diet." Diabetics are told to try to cut down on sugar, but to base their meals on starchy foods such as potatoes, rice, and pasta. Bread is encouraged, as are breakfast cereals.

I was recently in a London teaching hospital, chatting to a fifty-five-year-old man who was about to have his leg amputated because of type 2 diabetes. When I asked him what he was offered for breakfast, he said, "I had a choice of white bread or cornflakes."

Twenty years ago you could have been forgiven for feeding diabetics this sort of food. But since then there have been literally dozens of studies that have shown again and again that this is not the way to go.

A recent review of twenty randomized controlled trials involving over more than three thousand type 2 diabetics found that for losing weight, improving cholesterol num-

What Is the Mediterranean Diet?

The Mediterranean diet has become incredibly popular ever since studies showed it can significantly cut your risk of heart disease, type 2 diabetes, and possibly Alzheimer's. It is a diet that emphasizes the importance of eating fruit, vegetables, oily fish, nuts, and olive oil. Yogurt and cheese are warmly embraced, as is a glass of red wine at the end of the day (though this is optional). There are carbs in this diet, but the sort that your body takes longer to break down and absorb. That means legumes (beans and lentils), not pasta, rice, or potatoes. I think it is a fantastically healthful and tasty way to eat. It takes many of the best features of a low-carb diet and makes them more palatable. I go into much more detail about how to Mediterraneanize your diet later in the book. Indeed, it is the crux of the Blood Sugar Diet.

bers, and improving blood sugar control, the best bet is the low-carb Mediterranean diet. It's a diet that is moderately high in fat and low in highly processed carbohydrates.[19]

Dr. Unwin's Eureka Moment

After thirty years as a family doctor, David Unwin had become increasingly puzzled and gloomy about his patients. "I couldn't understand why more and more of them were coming into the office overweight and with type 2 diabetes, sometimes decades earlier than they used to," he explains. "I didn't know how to help them. More often than not I started them on medication."

Then one day a female patient turned up diabetes-free. "She mystified me. But I am always fascinated by stories of success, so I asked her what she had done."

She replied, "You're not going to like this, Doctor." She told him she had read about the benefits of a low-carb, high-fat diet and given it a try.

Dr. Unwin did some research and soon became convinced that part of the problem for type 2 diabetics is their metabolism can no longer deal with sugar. "It's become almost like a poison," he says. The obvious answer is to cut back, not just on sugar but also on foods that rapidly turn into sugars when they enter your body.

Putting patients on a low-carb diet is still viewed by many doctors as verging on the faddish, so it was against the advice of colleagues that he decided to do a small trial. He recruited nineteen patients who had type 2 diabetes or prediabetes and gave them a very simple diet sheet.

"Reduce starchy carbohydrates a lot (remember they are just concentrated sugar)," it reads. "If possible, cut out the white stuff like bread, pasta, rice. As for sugar, cut it out altogether, although it will be in the blueberries, strawberries, and raspberries you are allowed to eat freely."

Instead, patients were encouraged to eat more protein, butter, full-fat yogurt, and olive oil: "EATING LOTS OF VEGETABLES WITH PROTEIN AND FATS LEAVES YOU FULL IN A WAY THAT LASTS," he wrote in capital letters.

In a spirit of solidarity, and because he wanted to lose some weight himself, Dr. Unwin went on the diet. His wife, a clinical psychologist, worked with patients on the emotional aspects of weight loss. Crucially, rather than focusing on the downsides to type 2 diabetes, she helped patients to focus on the positive aspects of losing weight.

One of the patients dropped out early on, but the others found it simple and easy to stick to. They started out at an average weight of 220 pounds and over the eight months of the trial lost an average of more than 20 pounds, much of it around the waist.[20] Seven patients were able to come off medication, and most reported improved energy and well-being, which in turn meant they were more inclined to exercise. By the end only two of the nineteen still had raised blood sugars, and even those two had seen a huge improvement. There were also big improvements in blood pressure and cholesterol levels, despite the fact that his patients were now eating far more eggs and butter.

Dr. Unwin was struck by just how excited his patients were to take control of their own lives and not rely on him to solve their problems. People who were not officially part of the trial asked to join in.

"I was worried what other doctors in the practice would think," he says, looking back. "I thought they might think I was buying into something that was seen as mumbo-jumbo. But the success of the patients emboldened me."

The patients who lost the weight have kept it off, and more patients have gone through his program. "It is all about seeing the potential in people, giving them a choice," says Dr. Unwin.

Do You Crave Carbs? Are You Addicted?

Try this short quiz about your relationship to carbohydrates.

1. Do you get an instant reward or "hit" as soon as you eat sweet, starchy, or refined foods? **YES / NO**

2. Do you eat five or more portions of carbohydrates most days (in addition to sweet things, this includes pasta, bread, potatoes, rice, and cereals)? **YES / NO**

3. Do you often drink sweetened or flavored drinks (including fruit juice and artificially sweetened drinks)? **YES / NO**

4. Do you often snack or graze between meals?
   YES / NO

5. Do you eat three or more portions of fruit a day?
   YES / NO

6. Do you usually have generous portions of carbohydrate-rich foods with most of your meals, getting over 30 percent of your calories from starchy and/or refined carbohydrates, including bread, pasta, potatoes, rice, and cereals? (Whole-grain versions of all these still count as starch.) **YES / NO**

7. Do you often eat to make yourself feel better, such as when you are disappointed, are under pressure, or have had an argument? **YES / NO**

8. Are you eating large portions? **YES / NO**

9. Do you often feel unsatisfied, even soon after finishing a meal? **YES / NO**

10. Does the sight, smell, or thought of food often stimulate you to eat, even if you have just finished a meal or are not hungry? **YES / NO**

11. Do you often lose control and eat much more than you meant to, particularly when eating snacks, junk food, or sweets? (May involve eating until uncomfortable, feeling sick, or actually being sick.) **YES / NO**

12. Do you often justify eating by thinking, "Just this time" or "Later I will eat better/start the diet/burn it off"? **YES / NO**

13. Is food often on your mind? Do you frequently find yourself thinking about food during the day? **YES / NO**

14. Do you sometimes eat in secret?   **YES / NO**

15. Do you sometimes snack late in the evening or during the night?   **YES / NO**

16. Do you often feel guilty or ashamed about what you are eating, yet find yourself eating it again soon after?   **YES / NO**

17. Do you often crave carbohydrates or feel shaky, irritable, anxious, or sweaty without them?
YES / NO

RESULTS: Add up the number of yes answers and see which group you are in below.

0–3 You don't appear to be addicted. You can take it or leave it when it comes to eating carbs and probably have a fairly healthy attitude toward food.

4–8 You may be addicted to carbs. You like your carbs, but are probably managing to keep it in check. This may require a certain amount of self-control. At times you probably find this a bit of a challenge. The problem with carbs can be that the more you eat, the more you want. It is a slippery slope.

9–13 Moderately addicted to carbs. You are eating considerably more than you know is good for you and probably feeling bad about it. You are likely to be feeling hungry much of the time, preoccupied by food, and at times struggling to control your cravings as a result of a degree of insulin resistance. You are probably at risk of developing diabetes, if you don't have it already (even in the early stages). Worth getting regular health checks.

14–17 Severe addiction to carbs. Avoiding carbs is a real challenge for you. You are likely to be constantly hungry, preoccupied with food, feeling bad, and feeling guilty about your eating. You are highly likely to have insulin resistance (metabolic syndrome). Given the amount of carbs you are eating and your unhealthy relationship to carbohydrates, you're at significant risk of developing diabetes, if you don't have it already. Definitely worth getting regular health checks.

The Truth About Carbohydrates

I'm not saying all carbs are bad. Along with fats and proteins, carbs play an important role in our diet. The problem occurs when you eat too much of the wrong sort. Carbs broadly come in two main categories:

1. **Easily digestible carbs.** This is the kind that is rapidly absorbed by your body and creates an instant spike in blood sugar. This category includes not just the granulated sugar you add to your coffee or quaff down in sodas but also "natural" sweeteners such as honey, maple syrup, and agave nectar. Processed foods are stuffed full of sugars. Easily digestible carbs also include starches such as

bread, rice, pasta, and potatoes. This doesn't mean that rice and potatoes are evil, but don't pile your plate with them. Think of them more as a side dish than a staple, and try to find alternatives.

2. **Complex, unrefined carbs.** This is the "good" type of carbs, as they contain lots of fiber, making them harder to absorb. Slow absorption is a good thing. Examples include vegetables, legumes, and whole grains. Unfortunately, genuine, unprocessed whole grains are hard to find. While some breads and cereals may say "made with whole grains" on the package, many of these are in fact heavily processed or contain added sugars.

Easily digestible carbs are the baddies because they can cause blood sugar spikes and result in the overproduction of insulin. But how can you tell whether you are eating good or bad carbs?

One way is by looking up a food's glycemic index (GI). Unrefined carbohydrates normally have a low GI, meaning they cause blood sugar levels to rise slowly; that helps you to feel fuller for longer. Refined carbohydrates, on the other hand, tend to have a high GI, which means they cause a rapid spike in blood sugar levels, which then crash. This will encourage you to eat more.

GI is a measure of the speed at which your blood sugars rise. Foods are ranked from 0 to 100 (with sugar being 100). But the size of the spike in blood sugar and how long it stays high is a result not just of the type of food you eat but also of the amount of the carbs in that food. The way to measure the overall impact of a particular food on your blood sugar is by calculating its glycemic load (GL).

$$GL = (GI \times \text{the amount of carbohydrate}) \div 100$$

An apple, for example, has a GI of 40. It contains about 15 grams of carbs, so its glycemic load is:

$$GL = (40 \times 15) \div 100 = 6$$

If you think this sounds complicated, you're right—it is. To properly get your head around it I recommend going to the website of the University of Sydney, which has been at the forefront of GI research for over twenty years: www.glycemicindex.com.

The Sydney researchers say that, as a rule of thumb, you should be wary of carbs with a GI over 55 or a GL over 20. Foods with a high GI/GL include white bread, cornflakes, white rice, potatoes, and bagels. Those with a low GI/GL include most vegetables, nuts, seeds, certain whole grains, mushrooms, and most fruits.

See page 75 for a few examples.

As you can see, some of the foods that in the past we've been urged to fill up on, such as pasta and rice, have a very high GL. Switching to lower-GL versions of these staples can produce significant improvements in blood sugar control.

GI and GL are useful, but only up to a point. Trying to base what you eat entirely on glycemic index charts will prove stressful and complicated because, among other things, they

Food	Glycemic Index (GI) Under 55 is low	Glycemic Load Over 20 is high
Cooked carrots	33	2
Lentils	22	4
Apple	40	6
Apple juice	44	13
Mashed potato	83	17
White pasta (cooked)	61	29
Whole-grain pasta (cooked)	58	29
White rice	72	30
Brown rice	48	20
Bagel	69	24

don't take into account two other hugely important food groups, fats and proteins. I prefer a much simpler approach, which I detail later.

A Word on Fructose

One form of sugar that has been demonized above all others in recent years is fructose. So what is it, and why does it have such a bad reputation?

Fructose is a form of sugar that is commonly found in fruit and in ordinary table sugar. It is, notoriously, also found in high-fructose corn syrup, which has in the last few decades been added to many processed foods and carbonated drinks.

Fructose is incredibly sweet, but the main problem with it is the way it is treated by the body. Unlike glucose, which can be taken up by any cell, fructose has to be processed by the liver. In small amounts that is fine, but in the quantities we tend to consume today it leads to liver overload. One of the things that the liver does with excess fructose is turn it into fat. Load the liver with enough fructose and you get a fatty liver.

To cut down on fructose you will need to cut down on the sweet stuff—that is, sugar-sweetened drinks, many breakfast cereals, pastries, and desserts.

As noted above, fruit also contains fructose. And while it is good to consume a certain amount of fresh fruit, whole and where possible with the skin on, you should try to minimize your consumption of juices, which have had the fiber stripped out. A small glass of orange juice has twice the sugar, twice the calories, and half the fiber of an orange.

So Fiber Is a Good Thing?

Yes, eating more fiber is one other way to slow the rate at which your body absorbs sugar. Lack of fiber in our diet is a leading cause of the current diabesity epidemic. The average adult eats about 15 grams of fiber a day, but you should be eating at least twice that. Studies suggest that contemporary hunter-gatherers (the closest analog we have to our ancient ancestors) eat at least 100 grams of fiber per day, maybe more.

Fiber not only slows the absorption of sugars but, because it passes largely undigested through your small intestine, provides food for the trillions of healthy bacteria that lurk in the large intestine. There are thousands of different species of bacteria living in your gut, as rich an ecosystem as you will find in a rain forest, and having the right mix is important for your health. Eating plenty of fiber helps the "good guys" thrive.

You can get reasonable amounts of fiber by eating more beans, peas, bulgur, artichokes, leafy green vegetables, broccoli, cauliflower, carrots, cabbage, oats, nuts, raspberries, blackberries, apples, and pears.

CHAPTER FIVE

The Return of the Very Low-Calorie Diet

HAVE EXPLAINED WHY CUTTING OUT EASILY DIGESTIBLE carbs will help reduce hunger and blood sugar surges. Now I want to address some of the anxieties you might have about rapid weight loss before going on to look at the Blood Sugar Diet itself.

Most of us have heard countless times that if you lose weight fast, you will put it all back on even faster. It is a key part of dieting folklore.

I heard a leading nutritionist on the radio the other day saying with complete confidence, "Very low-calorie diets are really bad for you and they don't work. There's absolutely no benefit to doing them or fasting or detoxing. It's just wishful thinking."

A few years ago I would have agreed, and if you had asked me what I thought of rapid weight loss, I would have said it was a terrible idea. Everyone knows, I'd have said, about the dangers of yo-yo dieting. Everyone knows that the only successful way to lose weight in the long run is to do it gradually, sensibly, cutting your calories slowly, aiming to lose around 1 to 2 pounds a week. But that was before I began to take a serious look at the science. And it turns out that much of what I used to accept as "proven" is actually based on myth.

There is certainly a rich history of faddish crash diets out there, from the lemonade fast to the cabbage soup diet. The latest versions include juicing and cleansing diets, promising you can lose "7 pounds in 7 days." Now, some of these diets do deliver impressive weight loss, at least initially. The problem is that most of them are so boring that they become impossibly difficult to sustain. What's more, some have inadequate protein in them, leading to muscle loss (you need to maintain your muscle mass to keep your metabolic rate up and to help mop up sugar surges).

The other problem is that the scale lies. Just as jockeys are able to shed pounds two days before a race by fasting, at the start of a very low-calorie diet what you are losing is mainly water, not fat. The initial results are fabulous, but when you stop, the water piles back on, and so does the weight.

One of the most notorious of the crash diets was the Last Chance Diet, promoted in the 1970s by osteopath Robert Linn. Linn, who at one point weighed 235 pounds, became interested in diets after developing heart palpitations in his midforties. He began experimenting with high-protein liquid diets, lost a lot of weight, and then started up a weight loss clinic. He subsequently published his book, which sold well over 2.5 million copies.

Along with his bestselling book you could also buy his miraculous "liquid protein diet," Prolinn. Prolinn provided less than 400 calories a day, but it really seemed to work. There were numerous personal endorsements by celebrities who assured the public that they could lose up to 10 pounds a week.

After initial success, however, things fell apart. There were reports of deaths associated with the Last Chance Diet, and the FDA was asked to investigate. Although some of the reported deaths seem to have occurred in people who already had advanced heart disease and might have died anyway, there was evidence in a few people that the diet itself might be causing damage to the heart through what was identified as "protein-calorie malnutrition."

The thing about protein is that it is not a source of fuel like fat or carbohydrates, but primarily a source of amino acids. Among other things, amino acids help build muscle; they are used as a source of fuel only when your fat and carbohydrate stores start to run down.

Unlike fat or carbohydrates, the body doesn't store protein. If you don't get enough in your diet, your body will break down your muscles to top up your amino acids. The longer you go without, the more damage you do. That is why it is so important that whatever diet you go on, you make sure that it is rich in high-quality protein.

The problem for Last Chance dieters who used Prolinn or

other copycat products was that the protein in those sachets came largely from collagen, a low-quality protein obtained from the tendons, ligaments, and skin of animals. Living on nothing but chemically predigested cowhide and tendons scavenged from slaughterhouse animals and then enhanced with artificial flavorings and sweeteners was never likely to end well.

Not surprisingly, the Last Chance Diet and others of its type have cast a long shadow over the reputation of very low-calorie diets. But as some of America's leading obesity experts pointed out in a review article in the *New England Journal of Medicine* in 2013 (an article that is really worth reading), the belief that slow and gradual weight loss is more effective than rapid weight loss is a myth, despite the fact that it has been repeated in textbooks for decades.[21]

The authors point out that numerous trials have shown that "more rapid and greater initial weight loss is associated with lower body weight at the end of long-term follow-up." In other words, if you want to diet successfully it can be better to lose weight fast than slowly.

A recent Australian study backs up these claims.[22] Researchers took two hundred obese volunteers and put half of them on a very low-calorie diet (less than 800 calories a day). The goal was for these participants to lose 12.5 percent of their body weight within twelve weeks. The other participants were put on a low-fat diet, cutting their normal weekly intake by about 500 calories a day. They were given thirty-six weeks to achieve similar levels of weight loss as the faster dieters.

There was a very high drop-out rate among the steady low-fat dieters: less than half made it to the end of the thirty-six weeks. It's not surprising. Going low-fat is hard, and people often get frustrated by the slow rate of progress. By comparison, more than 80 percent of people assigned to the rapid weight loss program achieved their goal. On the downside, one person in the rapid weight group developed acute cholecystitis (inflammation of the gallbladder), which may have been due to the diet.

Katrina Purcell, a dietician who led the study, said, "Across the world, guidelines recommend gradual weight loss for the treatment of obesity, reflecting the widely held belief that fast weight loss is more quickly regained. However, our results show that achieving a weight loss target of 12.5 per cent is more likely, and drop-out is lower, if losing weight is done quickly." She thinks that losing weight fast motivates dieters to stick with their program because they see rapid results. A very low-calorie diet also means less carbohydrates, which forces the body to burn fat more quickly.

Both groups were then followed for another three years. Although most put back on some weight, it was similar amounts in both groups. Commenting on this study, Dr. Corby Martin and Dr. Kishore Gadde, from Pennington Biomedical Research Center in Baton Rouge, Louisiana, wrote, "This study . . . indicates that for weight loss, a slow and steady approach does not win the race, and the myth that rapid weight loss is associated with rapid weight regain is no more true than Aesop's fable."

Dr. Nick Finer, an endocrinologist and bariatric physician

at University College London Hospitals, also commented: "This study shows clearly that rapid weight loss does not lead to faster weight regain, but importantly can be a better approach since more people achieved their target loss, and fewer dropped out of treatment. If we couple these findings with those from other groups that have shown dramatic and immediate improvements in diabetes and blood pressure with rapid weight loss . . . this should be part of [our] approaches to treatment."

Dr. Taylor says there is a world of difference between a crash diet and what he's recommending. "A crash diet has an unplanned element to it: where you desperately cut out all food and only drink green juice before going back to what you did before. That is an unplanned crash. We have a planned approach to eating. Reduce food intake. Keep it low for eight weeks. Then have a stepped return to eating less than you used to. Often people want to keep dieting for longer. It is because they feel so well. Almost to a person, they say, 'I feel ten years younger.' What they are wary of is going back onto the stuff that used to poison them—too much food."

His colleague Dr. Mike Lean of Glasgow University is also adamant that for many people rapid weight loss is the way to go. "Doing it slowly is a torture. Contrary to the belief of dieticians, people who lose weight more quickly, more emphatically, are more likely to keep it off in the long term. Dieticians are still teaching that you should lose weight slowly to keep it off. Wrong. Wrong. Wrong. This is based largely on the very old 1960s low-calorie diet—people who went on crash diets with no maintenance program. If you have no maintenance program, of course you put the weight back on."

There are people who should be cautious about doing such a low-calorie diet, and I list them in the "Before You Start" section on page 102. But for many it could prove a pathway back to health.

Other Common Myths About Rapid Weight Loss

One myth heard very often is, "There's no point in doing a rapid weight loss diet because within a few days of starting you will go into starvation mode, your metabolic rate slows, and weight loss stops." False.

Fear of going into "starvation mode" is common and seems to be based, in part, on the Minnesota starvation experiment, carried out during World War II. In this study, thirty-six male volunteers spent six months on a low-calorie diet consisting largely of potatoes, turnips, bread, and macaroni.[23] The study was done to help scientists understand how to treat victims of mass starvation in Europe. Not fat to begin with, the volunteers became incredibly skinny and their metabolic rates slowed down. As you can see, however, this was an extreme situation.

A more recent experiment on the effects of short-term calorie restriction produced very different results. In this study, eleven healthy volunteers were asked to live on nothing but water for eighty-four hours (just under four days).[24] The researchers found that the volunteers' metabolic rate actually went *up* while they were fasting. By Day 3 it had risen, on average, by 14 percent. One reason for this may have been the rise in hormones known to burn fat.

In the long run your metabolic rate will slow down no matter how quickly or slowly you lose weight, simply because you are now no longer carrying the equivalent of a large, heavy suitcase full of fat wherever you go. That is why it is important to keep your metabolic rate up by doing strength exercises (which I'll talk about later) and keeping active as your weight drops.

A second myth heard quite often is, "It is better to set realistic weight loss goals, because if you are too ambitious you are doomed to fail." False.

We're always told to be realistic, and many people would say that trying to lose a lot of weight really fast is unrealistic. Yet research suggests that people who set out with more ambitious goals tend to lose more weight. In a study, nearly two thousand overweight men and women were asked about their goals before they started on a weight loss program.[25] They were followed for two years, by which time those with "less realistic goals" had lost the most weight.

A third common myth is, "If I cut my calories dramatically, I will feel hungry all the time and end up abandoning the diet." False.

Many of the people I've talked to who have done a very low-calorie diet say that hunger typically disappears within forty-eight hours. Some people get problems such as headaches, but these are often due to dehydration. You are missing out on the fluid you would normally take in with your food, plus as you burn fat you lose water. If you don't drink enough, your blood pressure can drop and you may feel faint. To anticipate and avoid this you should increase your fluid intake; I will write more on this in the next chapter.

Day One

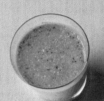

Breakfast: Blueberry and green tea smoothie (see page 174).

Lunch: Pepper with jeweled feta (see page 183).

Dinner: Eggplant with lamb and pomegranate (see page 201).

Calories: 810

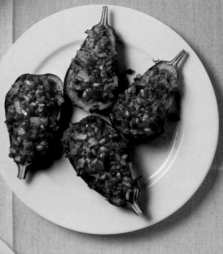

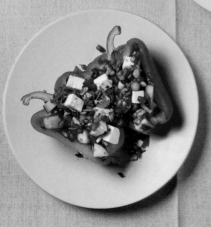

Day Two

Breakfast: Poached egg and avocado (see page 212).

Lunch: No-carb ploughman's (see page 214).

Dinner: Vegetable curry with cauliflower rice (see pages 219–20).

Calories: 790

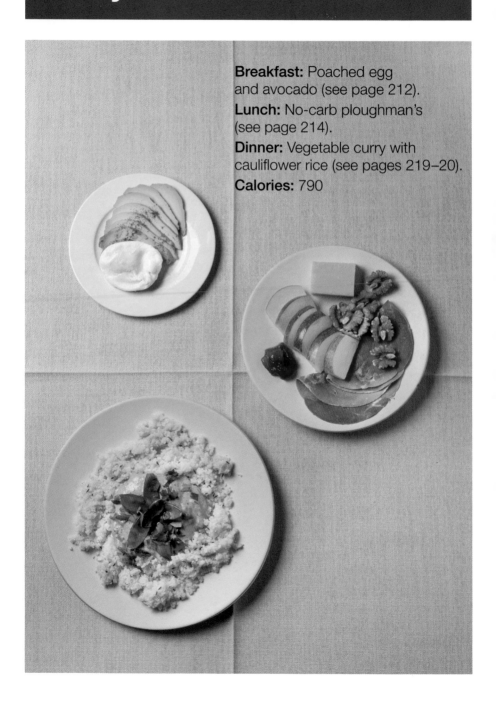

Day Three

Breakfast: No-carb muesli (see page 171).
Lunch: Beet falafel (see page 182).
Dinner: Vegetable frittata (see page 175).
Calories: 790

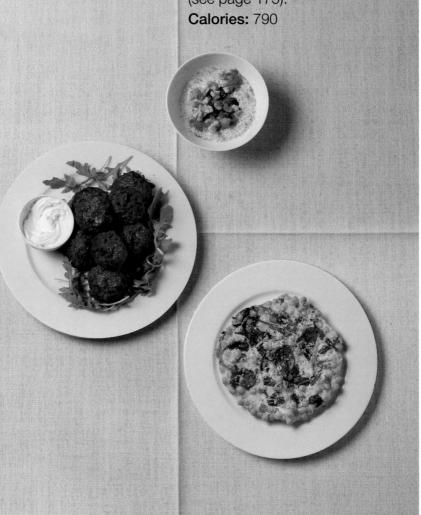

Day Four

Breakfast: Portobello "toast" with goat cheese and pine nuts (see page 171).

Lunch: Sardine dip (see page 214).

Dinner: Foil-steamed fish (see page 207).

Calories: 840

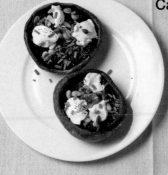
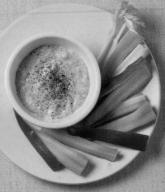
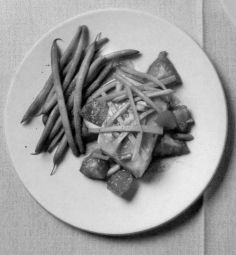

Day Five

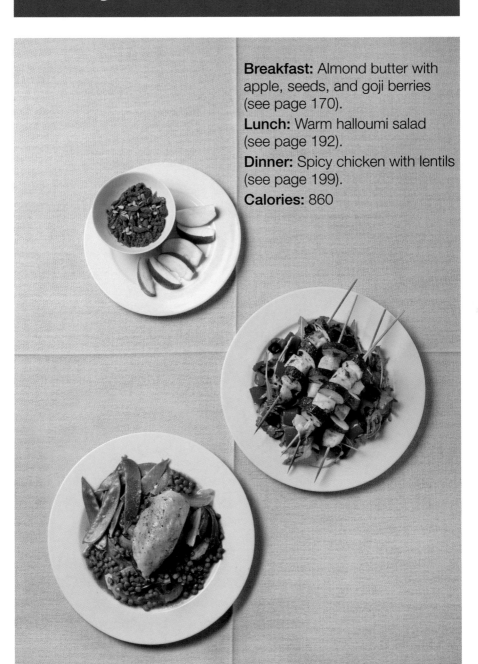

Breakfast: Almond butter with apple, seeds, and goji berries (see page 170).

Lunch: Warm halloumi salad (see page 192).

Dinner: Spicy chicken with lentils (see page 199).

Calories: 860

Day Six

Brunch: Poached egg and smoked salmon stack (see page 177).

Dinner: Harissa chicken (see page 203).

Calories: 740

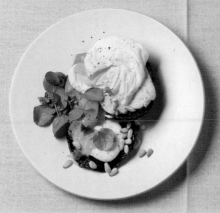

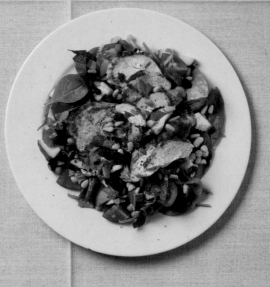

Day Seven

Brunch: Cheesy baked beans (see page 214).
Dinner: Steak with crème fraîche and peppercorn sauce (see page 202).
Calories: 770

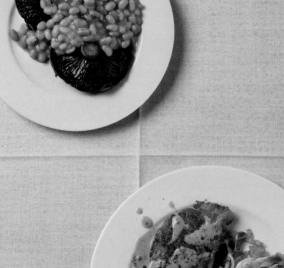

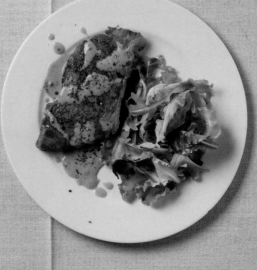

Quick Soups

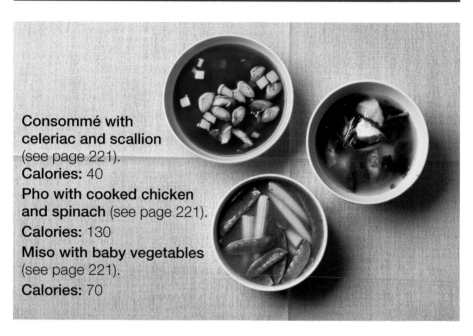

Consommé with celeriac and scallion (see page 221).
Calories: 40

Pho with cooked chicken and spinach (see page 221).
Calories: 130

Miso with baby vegetables (see page 221).
Calories: 70

Blood Sugar Diet **favorite ingredients**

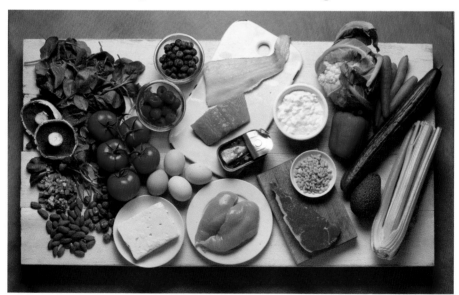

The Blood Sugar Diet

The Three Core Principles of the Blood Sugar Diet and What to Do Before You Start

S O FAR I'VE EXPLAINED THE BACKGROUND TO THE current obesity crisis, underlined the dangers that come with prediabetes and diabetes, introduced you to the science behind the very low-calorie diet approach, and, I hope, inspired you with stories of people who have already done it.

Now it's time to get on to the practicalities of the diet itself. It is a bold and radical diet, one that involves eating 800 calories a day for up to eight weeks. It will help you get rid of your visceral (abdominal) fat fast. Once your visceral fat levels start to drop (and this happens within days), then the fat clogging up your liver will also begin to melt away like snow under a hot sun. Within weeks both prediabetics and type 2 diabetics should see their blood sugar levels falling back toward normal. This will set you on course for a leaner, healthier future.

But this is not just a one-off weight loss program, something you do for a few weeks and then are done with forever. It is part of a lifestyle system built on three core principles that are intended to support you not only while you are on the diet but also, crucially, when you have finished and are moving on to the next stage in your life. Understanding and applying these principles is important for long-term success. So here they are, the three core principles of the Blood Sugar Diet: going Mediterranean, getting active, and sorting out your head.

1. Going Mediterranean

I am going to introduce you to a Mediterranean-style low-carb eating plan. This is a tasty and healthy way of living. It is low in starchy, easily digestible carbs, but packed full of disease-fighting vitamins and flavonoids. It is rich in olive oil, fish, nuts, fruit, and vegetables, but also contains lots of delicious foods that over the years we have been told not to eat, such as full-fat yogurt and eggs.

In huge, randomized studies researchers have found not only that people get multiple health benefits from a Mediterranean style of eating but also that it's easy and enjoyable to stick to (unlike a low-fat diet).[26]

Although it is derived from the eating habits of people living in Mediterranean countries, you can apply the principles of Mediterranean-style eating to a wide range of different cuisines, from Chinese and Indian to Mexican and Scandinavian.

2. Getting Active

We all know how important being more active is, yet few of us find the time or inclination to go on regular runs or visit the gym. If you are thinking, "You must be joking—I can't possibly become more active while cutting my calories," then be reassured that the activity program I outline in Chapter Eight is not going to leave you tired or hungry. It should improve your mood and make the diet easier. Being more active is also the best way to reverse insulin resistance, which lies at the heart of most blood sugar problems.

In brief, you will start by standing up more (later on I will go into the science of why simply getting up every thirty minutes for one minute or so makes such a big difference). Everyone can do this.

You will need to increase the amount that you walk. In "Before You Start" (see page 102), I will give you a simple way to assess your current level of fitness.

You will also need to embark on a set of strength-building resistance exercises, which you will start on Day 1 of the diet and build over the eight weeks. No special equipment is required.

Finally, you will be introduced to one of the biggest breakthroughs in sports science in the last decade. It is a cardio program that in a few weeks can significantly improve your aerobic fitness, the strength of your heart and lungs. The program outlined in this book has been specifically designed for diabetics and those who are currently not very fit, and you will be pleased to hear that it does not involve hours of jogging. In fact, it requires only a few minutes a week. It is optional, but it is very effective, and it is something I now do on a regular basis.

3. Sorting Out Your Head

The last of the three core principles is about getting your head in the right place—learning how to de-stress and reduce impulsive eating.

We all know how easy it is when things go wrong to reach for the cookies or cake. Well, this is the stress hormone, cortisol, in action. As well as driving "comfort eating," cortisol makes your body more insulin-resistant, which makes you hungry. All good reasons to get your stress levels down.

While making a science documentary about the brain not long ago, *The Truth About Personality*, I investigated different ways to reduce stress and build resilience, and the one that I found most effective was mindfulness. It's a modern take on meditation, something that has been practiced by all the great religions. In recent years mindfulness has become incredibly fashionable among celebrities, business leaders, and athletes. The reason is that it works. A few short sessions of mindfulness done each week should be enough to reduce stress and anxiety.[27] I was skeptical before I began doing it three years ago, but I have now made it part of my life.

So these are the three core principles that will support you through the Blood Sugar Diet and which I hope you'll maintain when you finish it. Because it is so important to what comes next, I am going to spell out how to Mediterraneanize your eating habits before moving on to the details of the Blood Sugar Diet as a whole.

The "M Plan"

There have been numerous studies that provide overwhelming evidence of the benefits of Mediterranean-style eating, one of the most impressive being the PREDIMED trial (Prevención con Dieta Mediterránea), which began in 2003 and is still ongoing. For this trial Spanish researchers recruited more than 7,400 people, many of them type 2 diabetics, and randomly assigned them to either a Mediterranean diet or a low-fat diet.[28]

Both groups were encouraged to eat lots of fresh fruit, vegetables, and legumes (beans, lentils, and peas). They were also discouraged from consuming sugary drinks, cakes, sweets, or pastries and from eating too much processed meat (such as bacon or salami).

The main difference between the two diets was that those assigned to the Mediterranean diet were asked to eat plenty of nuts and oily fish; they were told to use lots of olive oil and allowed to enjoy the occasional glass of wine with their evening meal. They were also encouraged to eat plenty of eggs, plus some chocolate (preferably dark, with more than 50 percent cacao content). The low-fat group, by contrast, was encouraged to eat low-fat dairy products

What Is Your M Score?

(Adapted from R. Estruch et al., "Primary Prevention of Cardiovascular Disease with a Mediterranean Diet," *New England Journal of Medicine*, April 4, 2013.)

Add 1 point for each yes answer. A total of 10 or more is good.

1. Do you use olive oil as your main fat for cooking and salad dressings?

2. Do you eat 2 or more servings of vegetables a day? (1 serving = 7 ounces; potatoes do not count as a vegetable)

3. Do you eat 2 or more servings of fruit a day? (No points for sweet tropical fruits such as melons, grapes, pineapples, and bananas, however.)

4. Do you eat less than 1 serving of processed meat (ham, bacon, sausage, salami) a day? (1 serving = 3½ ounces)

and consume lots of starchy foods, such as bread, potatoes, pasta, and rice.

The result? Well, it turned out that those on the Mediterranean diet were 30 percent less likely to die from a heart attack or stroke. Subsequent studies have shown even more health benefits (more on these shortly).

Dr. Mario Kratz, a nutritional scientist at the Fred Hutchinson Cancer Research Center in Seattle who has

5. Do you eat full-fat yogurt at least three times a week?

6. Do you eat 3 or more servings of legumes (peas, beans, lentils) a week? (1 serving = 5¼ ounces)

7. Do you eat 3 or more servings of whole grains a week? (1 serving = 5¼ ounces)

8. Do you eat oily fish, shrimp, or shellfish 3 or more times a week? (1 serving = 3½ to 5¼ ounces)

9. Do you eat sweet treats such as cakes, cookies, etc., less than 3 times a week?

10. Do you eat 1 serving of nuts (1 serving = 1 ounce) 3 or more times a week?

11. Do you cook with garlic, onions, and tomatoes at least 3 times a week?

12. Do you average around 7 glasses of wine or spirits a week? (Much more than 7 glasses can be harmful.)

13. Do you sit at the table to eat at least twice a day?

14. Do you drink sodas less than once a week?

looked at lots of studies on low-fat versus high-fat dairy, says, "None of the research suggests low-fat dairy is better." In fact plenty of studies have found that eating full-fat dairy is *less* likely to lead to obesity.[29]

The impressive thing about the Mediterranean diet is just how widespread its benefits are. Not only does it cut your risk of heart disease and diabetes,[30] but a very recent finding is that women who ate a Mediterranean diet had 68 percent less chance of developing breast cancer than those on a low-fat diet.[31] Consuming extra-virgin olive oil seems to be particularly beneficial when it comes to helping prevent cancer, perhaps because it contains compounds such as polyphenols, which are known to be anti-inflammatory.

Tip: Keep your oils in a cupboard,
as they degrade in sunlight.

The Mediterranean diet even seems to keep your brain in better shape. Again, studies show that those assigned to a Mediterranean diet were less likely, as they got older, to develop dementia or cognitive impairment (that's when you struggle to learn new things, remember, or make decisions) than those trying to eat a low-fat diet.[32]

Finally, a brief note on alcohol. The Mediterranean diet includes a glass of wine with the evening meal. There have been endless arguments as to whether drinking moderate amounts of alcohol is healthful or not. The best way to find out would be to give alcohol to a group of nondrinkers and see what happens. Well, a research team in Israel has recently done just that.[33] They took 224 diabetics who did not drink and randomly assigned them to drinking a medium-sized glass (5 fluid ounces) of either red wine, white wine, or mineral water for their evening meal, every evening, for two years.

So what happened? Well, red wine drinkers will be delighted to hear it was the group drinking red wine who came out on top. They saw significant improvements in their cholesterol levels and the quality of their sleep. Some also had better blood sugar control.

Based on all of the above, I've come up with a very simple one-page guide on how to Mediterraneanize your diet, which diabetic and prediabetic patients have tried with considerable success.

What's rather depressing is that although most doctors are aware of the research I've just quoted, many don't feel comfortable putting it into practice. A recent survey of 236 cardiologists and internal medicine physicians at a large U.S. academic medical center found that while all of them think nutrition is important, only 13 percent felt sufficiently well informed to talk to patients about it. Most admitted to spending less than three minutes per visit advising their patients about diet or exercise.[34]

Again, though most of them knew that a Mediterranean diet can cut the risk of heart disease and stroke, few were aware that in randomized trials low-fat diets have failed to

The M Plan: What to Eat to Control Your Weight and Your Blood Sugar

First, cut down on sugar, sugary treats, sugary drinks, and sugary desserts. No more than once or twice a week and preferably less. We offer lots of recipes for healthy alternatives later in the book. You can use sugar substitutes like stevia and xylitol, but try to wean yourself off your sweet tooth.

Minimize or avoid the starchy white stuff. Avoid white bread, pasta, potatoes, and rice. Be wary of alternatives that say things like "made with whole grains": if it's not 100 percent whole grain, the extra fiber can be negligible, and some whole-grain breads have added sugar. Brown rice is okay. Other good choices include quinoa, bulgur (cracked wheat), whole rye, whole barley, wild rice, and buckwheat. Legumes (lentils, beans, and peas) are healthful and filling.

Avoid most breakfast cereals. They are usually full of sugar, even the ones that contain bran.

Oatmeal is good, as long as it is not the instant sort.

Full-fat yogurt is also good. For flavor, add berries, such as blackberries, strawberries, or blueberries, or a sprinkling of nuts.

Start the day with eggs. Boiled, poached, scrambled, or as an omelet, eggs will keep you fuller for longer than cereal or toast. Delicious with smoked salmon, mushrooms, and a sprinkle of chili powder.

Snack on nuts. They are a great source of protein and fiber. Try to avoid salted or sweetened nuts, as they can encourage you to overdo it.

Eat more healthful fats and oils. Along with oily fish (salmon, tuna, mackerel), consume more olive oil. A splash makes vegetables taste better and improves the absorption of certain vitamins. Use olive oil, canola oil, or coconut oil for cooking.

Avoid margarine. Use butter instead. Cheese in moderation is fine.

Choose high-quality proteins. Top choices include oily fish, shrimp, chicken, turkey, pork, beef, and eggs. Other protein-rich foods include soy, edamame, Quorn meat substitute products, and hummus. Processed meats (ham, bacon, salami, sausage) should be eaten only a few times a week.

Eat plenty of different-colored vegetables. Mix it up, including everything from dark leafy greens to bright red and yellow peppers. Add sauces and flavoring: lemon, butter or olive oil, salt, pepper, garlic, chili, gravy.

Avoid too many sweet fruits. Berries, apples, or pears are fine, but sweet tropical fruits such as mangoes, pineapples, melons, and bananas are full of sugar.

Have a drink, but not too much. Try not to average more than one drink a day (one drink is a small glass of wine or one shot of spirits). Minimize beer, which is rich in carbs.

do so, which may be why so many still recommend a low-fat diet.

As the Harvard School of Public Health points out on its website, the final nail in the low-fat coffin should have been the Women's Health Initiative (WHI) Dietary Modification Trial.[35] In this trial, which began in 1993, 48,000 women were randomly assigned to either a low-fat diet or a control group that continued to eat normally. After eight years the trial was stopped. There were no differences in rates of cancer, heart disease, or weight between the two groups.

This is not a license to guzzle pints of cream and have lots of fried food, but it does mean that healthful fats such as olive oil and nuts can be eaten without guilt.

Before You Start

Confucius, the Chinese philosopher, pointed out more than two thousand years ago: "Success depends upon previous preparation, and without such preparation there is sure to be failure." Or as the actor Will Smith put it more recently, "I've always considered myself to be just average talent and what I have is a ridiculous, insane obsessiveness for practice and preparation."

The first thing I recommend you do is read this book all the way through to the end. The temptation is to dive into the plan, but it is important to get a full overview before you start. It is also important to be able to explain to your doctor what it is you are trying to achieve and the science behind it.

Talk to Your Doctor

I've been a bit critical about doctors in the early section of this book, but I am not anti-doctor, by any means. Most are very open-minded. Some of my best friends are doctors. I'm married to one. My son is training to become one. So do talk to yours before starting.

If you are on medication, it is particularly important to have your physician's buy-in, as he or she should be involved in monitoring you and tapering off your medication as needed. While many doctors will be delighted that you are taking responsibility for your health, some may be unimpressed. If yours is in that group, work on him or her. Make a bet with your doctor that you will succeed. It will give you motivation. And your success may inspire your doctor to recommend it to other patients.

Caution—make sure you discuss your plan with your doctor if any of the following apply:

- ★ You have a history of eating disorders
- ★ You are on insulin or a diabetic medication other than metformin (you may need to plan a suitable reduction in medication to avoid too fast a drop in blood sugar)
- ★ You are on blood pressure medication (you may have to reduce the dose or come off it)
- ★ You have moderate or severe retinopathy (if so, you should have extra screening within six months of reducing blood sugar levels)

★ You are pregnant or breast-feeding

★ You have a significant psychiatric disorder

★ You are taking the blood thinner warfarin

★ You have some form of epilepsy

★ You have another significant medical condition

Don't do the diet if:

★ You are under eighteen years old

★ Your BMI is below 21

★ You are recovering from surgery or you are generally in poor health

The following is a link to the Newcastle University website where you can get useful information, including a fact sheet that Dr. Taylor has written for health care professionals and which you can download and give to your doctor: www.ncl.ac.uk/magres/research/diabetes/reversal.htm. As he points out, you should confirm with your doctor that you really are a type 2 diabetic. There are other, rarer forms of the disease, including pancreatogenic, monogenic, or slow-onset type 1 diabetes, that will not respond in the same way to weight loss.

Getting to Know Yourself: Tests You Should Have Done

I love finding out more about my own body, and I find it fascinating to monitor the changes that occur when I embark on a new exercise regime or try a new food. You can keep records of your results in a diary or log in to thebloodsugardiet .com, where you can keep your data safely and anonymously. The site will also provide useful updates on the latest science and a wealth of other information.

Another reason to keep a diary, electronic or otherwise, is to monitor exactly what you eat and drink. Some of those who have successfully done this diet used the MyFitnessPal website or app to monitor calories and other nutrient intake. But a diary is only of value if it is honest and accurate. A few years ago I made a film where we asked an overweight actress to keep a food diary for a couple of weeks. At the same time we gave her a drink containing something called "doubly labeled water," which enabled us to estimate how many calories she was really consuming. When we added up the foods listed in her diary, it came to 1,500 calories, but the doubly labeled water technique suggested she was consuming far more than that. Before you tut-tut, remember that underestimating your calorie intake can happen quite easily.

The other bit of tech worth investing in is some way of tracking how many steps you do. This could be an app, a pedometer, or a Fitbit. You need to record how many steps you take on an average day before you start on the diet.

It's best to keep track during a typical week; the number is likely to be around 5,000. Whatever it is, I want you to write it down, and then aim to increase the number of steps you take by around 10 percent a week throughout the course of the diet. By the end I would hope you would be doing at least 10,000 steps, maybe more. I'll explain later why 10,000 steps is such an important figure.

Measure Your Pulse, Weight, and Waist

Find a quiet moment and take your pulse for sixty seconds. You will find it throbbing away on your wrist, just outside the outer-most tendon. Your pulse is a measure of your overall fitness. Measure it a few times, then write down the average number. I'd expect to see it improve over the coming few weeks.

Next I want you to weigh yourself. So head to the bathroom and onto the digital scale. With this number and your height, you can calculate your BMI. See the appendix at the back of the book for how to do this, or go to our website, www.thebloodsugardiet.com, which will do it automatically for you.

While you are in the bathroom, I want you to whip out a tape measure and measure your waist size. Honestly. There is no point in trying to hold everything in. You measure your waist size by going around your belly button; do not rely on your pants size (men typically underestimate their waist size by about 2 to 3 inches).

Why is waist size important? Because it is an indirect measure of your visceral fat and one of the best predictors we have of future health. As I've pointed out before, fat in and around the abdomen is dangerous even if you are not otherwise obviously overweight. Ideally your waist should be less than half your height. For example, if you are 6 feet tall, your waist should be less than 36 inches.

According to a recent survey of more than 32,000 American men and women,[36] waist sizes in the United States are expanding at a frightening rate. Between 2009 and 2011 the average American male's waist grew from 39 to nearly 40 inches; the average woman's belly expanded even more, from 36 to 38 inches. This is a whopping 12 inches more than average waist sizes in the 1950s. Marilyn Monroe, who had a 22-inch waist, was not exceptional for her time. Frank Hu, professor of nutrition and epidemiology at the Harvard School of Public Health, thinks that high-sugar diets and increased stress hormones may be largely responsible.

Now that you've noted your pulse, weight, and waist, take some selfies, or get a friend to take photos of you. Keep these pictures somewhere safe so you can compare the outward changes after you've done this diet. I predict that you will want to show people the "before" and "after" pictures.

Measure Your Fasting Glucose

This is a finger prick test you can do yourself (you can buy reliable digital blood sugar monitoring kits at drugstores and online), or you may prefer to ask your doctor. It should be done in the fasting state, that is, first thing in the morning, before breakfast, when you have been without food for at least eight hours. If the result is abnormal, you will need to repeat it and do further tests.

Normal range: 70 to 100 mg/dl (3.9 to 5.5 mmol/l)

Prediabetes: 101 to 125 mg/dl (5.6 to 7.0 mmol/l)

Diabetic: over 125 mg/dl (5.6 to 7.0 mmol/l)

There is disagreement about exactly where "normal" ends and prediabetes begins. The figures above are from the American Diabetes Association. The World Health Organization says "normal" is under 110 mg/dl (6.1 mmol/l), while the UK's National Institute for Health and Care Excellence recommends you keep the figure below 106 mg/dl (5.9 mmol/l).

Other routine tests you should ask your doctor about include A1C (a measure of blood sugar over the long term), a CBC (complete blood count), kidney function tests (urea and electrolytes), liver function tests (including GGT, a good measure of how healthy your liver is), and a blood lipids profile.

It would be more unusual to get your insulin levels measured, but if you do, your doctor will be able to calculate how insulin-resistant you are. I have included more details on all these in the Appendix.

Specialist Tests

The following tests are not routine, but they are revealing and can be highly motivating.

Dual-energy X-ray absorptiometry (DEXA) scan. This is used to measure visceral fat. By doing a DEXA scan at the start, another four weeks in, and a third at the end, you can track changes as you go along. It is more expensive but also more reliable than simply weighing yourself. Sticking DEXA images to your fridge door will remind you why you are doing this.

Liver ultrasound scan. Like the GGT blood test, this is a way of assessing the health of your liver. It will give you an estimate of how much fat you have in it.

Magnetic resonance imaging (MRI). This is the most accurate way of measuring liver and pancreatic fat, but it is time-consuming and expensive. If you want to see an MRI of my body when I was 20 pounds heavier and TOFI (thin on the outside, fat inside), then go to thebloodsugardiet.com. All that white stuff smothering my liver and pancreas is fat. Be warned: it's not pretty.

Kitchen Hygiene: Clear out Your Cupboards

If there are foods you want to avoid eating, don't keep them in the house. It might sound obvious, but if chocolatey or sugary snacks are right at hand, then unless you have superhuman willpower, there will come a time when you will eat them. My daughter has never forgiven me for eating her chocolate Easter egg when she was ten. It was sitting there, in full view. I couldn't resist taking a bite. Then another. Then it was all gone.

If you have children and feel you have to have sweet or salty treats in the house, then this makes things more difficult. If you are fortunate enough to have a partner who isn't a carb addict, get him or her to keep the treats in a locked cupboard. I'm not kidding. I sometimes have a bit of chocolate after a meal, but I get my wife to hide the bar; otherwise I would eat the whole thing. The safest course of action is to give it all away. The junk has to go. It will, however, leave space for healthier foods.

Write Down Your Goals

When you are working on establishing a new way of eating, you will inevitably have moments of doubt, when you forget why you are putting yourself through it. So, before you start, jot down all the reasons you want to get your blood sugar under control. Make them as specific as you can. Keep the list with you; maybe make it into your screen saver. Read this list whenever you feel yourself weakening.

Remember, you have really good reasons—what psychologists call a "driver"—to change. This isn't about vanity (though you will almost certainly look better). It isn't about what size your jeans are (though you should drop several sizes). It's about getting healthy. It's about getting your life back.

One of the goals you absolutely have to write down is how much weight you plan to lose. Any amount will help, particularly if you are in the prediabetes phase, but to properly reverse type 2 diabetes you will probably need to lose 10 to 15 percent of your current body weight. I lost 20 pounds, which was 11 percent of my body weight, and that for me did the trick. If your starting BMI is over 40, then you may need to lose more.

As I've mentioned before, we all have different personal fat thresholds—that is, the point at which fat begins to be stored in the liver and pancreas, affecting blood sugar levels. That's why it is important to know what's happening to your blood sugar while doing the diet. And for that reason I suggest you invest in a digital blood sugar monitor.

Find a Diet Buddy

Being part of a group—even if it's just you and one friend— will significantly improve your chances of success. We're planning to set up a place on thebloodsugardiet.com where people can form online groups for mutual support and encouragement. So do come along and help make it happen.

Once you've decided that you want to do this diet, tell your friends and family all about it. They may know someone else who wants to do it with you. The fact that you are making a public commitment also means you are more likely to stick to it.

When Should I Start?

The sooner the better. That said, you should find a period in your life where you know you can clear at least six weeks to focus on losing weight.

It's fine to keep working. In fact, keeping busy will help. But make sure your work colleagues are on board and not dumping doughnuts on your desk to "cheer you up." Likewise, you don't want your fiftieth birthday or your friend's wedding to derail you. By the same token, don't look for excuses not to start.

Once you've talked to your doctor, done your tests, cleared the junk food out of your cupboards, taped your goals to the fridge, and found a diet buddy, it's time to get going.

"Going on This Diet Is Like Preparing for an Expedition"

When Paul starts craving a sugary muffin for breakfast, he does something that might horrify you (it certainly horrifies him): he goes online and looks up pictures of feet just before they are about to be amputated. This is a man who is taking it seriously. Very seriously.

Paul—who describes himself as "a real foodie" and says that shopping for food, cooking, and eating are all great pleasures—asked his doctor to give him three months to try turning around his type 2 diagnosis before prescribing medication.

Soon after starting the diet, he began doing the training sessions I detail in this book—a workout for muscle building and an aerobic routine. He supplemented this routine with long walks and bicycle rides. Every morning he measured his blood sugar and wrote the results down in a notebook.

His advice? "It is like preparing for an expedition," he says. "You can't do it halfheartedly. You have to commit. It is like flicking a switch—you just have to say to yourself, 'I am not going to do anything that jeopardizes this.' "

Paul weighed 172 pounds when he was diagnosed. Like 35 percent of type 2 diabetics, his BMI was within the healthy range. However, he knew he was at risk: his mother is diabetic, and when he puts on weight it settles around his middle, which is a clear danger sign. "I was walking around with my head in the sand," he says. "I kept putting off addressing it."

Then two years ago his wife died from breast cancer (an emotional upheaval, as we have seen, is often part of the story). He started drinking more—and his weight crept up. Going on the diet was, in a way, a sign that it was time for a new chapter in his life to begin.

"It's a line in the sand. It has been very positive. It means that I want to take care of myself again. It means I have climbed out of a trough of despond and I am looking after myself. It's significant. A way of taking control again in a way that I had lost. To feel that I can—and want to—do this is empowering."

CHAPTER SEVEN

The Diet in Practice

YOU HAVE DECIDED TO GO FOR IT. YOU HAVE TALKED to your doctor, cleared your cupboards, and had some tests done. As you will soon discover, the Blood Sugar Diet isn't quite as tough as you may fear. Yes, you are going to be living on 800 calories a day for the next few weeks, but your body should adapt reasonably quickly. There is one final decision to make. Do you want to do the diet entirely with real food, or do you want to do it in part with commercial meal-replacement diet shakes?

Two Ways to Go

In Dr. Taylor's studies, largely for reasons of convenience, the subjects were asked to lose weight by drinking commercial meal-replacement diet shakes for the whole eight weeks, supplemented with some nonstarchy vegetables. If you are running a scientific study, then using diet shakes is not only convenient but also an easier way to keep close tabs on just how many calories people are actually consuming. But others have done it very successfully on real food. It's a personal decision. You have to decide which suits you best.

Meal-Replacement Shakes

If you decide to start with meal-replacement diet shakes, you should aim to consume around 600 calories per day in shakes, plus 200 calories' worth of nonstarchy vegetables. You will need that extra fiber from the vegetables (plus lots of water) to avoid getting constipated. We have provided some 200-calorie recipes—vegetable dishes and soups—in the recipe section later in the book.

The advantages of reputable meal-replacement diet shakes is that you know you are getting a balance of the right nutrients and you don't have to think about food. The disadvantage is that none of the commercial shakes I've tried so far have been particularly pleasant. I imagine that in time they would get boring.

I also think it is important, while you are on the diet, to learn how to cook proper, healthful, delicious meals. This will prepare you for life after the diet. A reasonable compromise might be to start with the shakes, get settled in, then after you have been on the diet for, say, two weeks, switch to eating mostly real food.

Real Food

Doing the diet with real food is slightly harder because you have to make sure that you are getting the right amount of protein, fat, vitamins, and other nutrients. That is why I asked Dr. Sarah Schenker, one of the United Kingdom's leading dieticians, to provide a range of simple, nutritious recipes, as well as a detailed and balanced dietary plan (see pages 167–225).

The principle behind the recipes is Mediterranean-style, low-carb eating. They are packed with nutrients and decent amounts of fats and protein; they are flavorsome and varied, so there is less chance that your taste buds will get bored and start craving the bad stuff.

If you want to do your own thing and make up your own Med-style, low-carb recipes, then do make sure that you are getting a varied diet with adequate amounts of the right nutrients. You may want to take a multivitamin pill to be on the safe side.

I think one of the other main advantages of doing this diet with real food is that this will retrain your taste buds. You may be someone who is not currently particularly fond of vegetables, but when you are on a low-calorie diet they will taste delicious! Remember, you are resetting your body not just for the next few months but hopefully for good.

Q & A

What does 800 calories look like?

More than you might think (check out the picture section in this book, where seven days' worth of 800 calories per day are laid out for you) but less than you're used to. The key to this diet is that every single mouthful packs a punch. And it scores high on what dieticians call the satiety factor—the feeling of fullness after eating that suppresses the urge to eat between meals. You should feel satisfied by smaller portions and won't stay forever hungry and preoccupied by food. As you watch the weight fall off you will get a lot of positive reinforcement to keep you going.

Why 800 calories? Why not eat more, or less?

If you have problems with blood sugar and want to regain your health, then you need to lose fat, particularly abdominal fat. It doesn't really matter how quickly or slowly you do it, but you may find it easier to lose it fast. Losing weight fast, if it's done properly, is motivating. Eight hundred calories is low, as diets go, but not super low.

There are carbohydrates in this diet, yet you say I shouldn't eat them.

There are some carbohydrates in the menus provided—but the right sort. As you will know by now, starchy carbohydrates are essentially concentrated sugars and are disruptive

exercise program will
essing from prediabe-
National Institutes of
thousand people with
rcent weight loss com-
he participants' risk of
er the next five years.[37]
on Program, visit www
.htm.

hat to Do
Expect

Weeks

nd that you begin to lose
, but initially you will also
ntial that you drink at least
ee fluid a day or you will
idaches. What you drink is
contain calories. It could be
ot thrilled with plain water,
ueeze of lemon or lime, or
e seltzer with lots of ice and
the occasional coffee (with
ople like drinking hot water;
ce that heat alone can soothe
as if you must. But avoid fruit

to blood sugar. You will find recipes here that include oats or brown rice—but in small quantities. It's a taste, not the main component of the meal. These carbohydrates are the slow-burning kind; they take time and energy to digest, which means you'll feel less hungry.

So what's going to keep me feeling full?

Fat and protein keep you feeling fuller for longer. The standard recommendations for protein are around 45 grams a day for a woman and 55 grams per day for a man. Good proteins to eat include eggs, fish, chicken, pork, shrimp, and tofu. Nuts, seeds, and legumes are packed full of protein too.

Is this a low-fat diet?

No—because, as I explained earlier, fat isn't the bad guy that it was once made out to be. It includes plenty of oily fish, a judicious amount of animal fat from meat, and plenty of plant fat (from nuts, seeds, olive oil, and avocados), as well as the fat in unsweetened yogurt. On the other hand, to lose weight fast you have to cut down on calories, so you won't find large amounts of cheese in the recipes.

Is snacking on fruit okay?

Fruit contains far more sugar than vegetables. There is some fruit in this diet, but it is rationed and used as an ingredient rather than an excuse to eat between meals. If you're looking for something to stir into yogurt, go for deep-colored blueberries, blackberries, cherries, or strawberries. But limit your intake of tropical fruit, which tends to be higher in

sugar. And steer clear of dates and other dried fruit—
two dates has the same effect on your blood sugar as
two large basketfuls of strawberries.

Are some vegetables better than others?

Absolutely. Vegetables contain much less sugar than fruit,
some are starchier than others, which means they will af
your blood sugar. Leafy green vegetables such as spinach, c
bage, lettuce, kale, and chard are rich in vitamin C and fil
and very low in sugar and starch, as are broccoli and cau
flower, so dig in. Ditto for tomatoes, cucumbers, and peppe
It gets more complicated with root vegetables such as pota
toes, parsnips, and turnips; these are quite high in starch, s
they should be treated with more caution.

Do I have to eat breakfast?

It's a myth that everyone has to eat breakfast. I love it, but
some people don't. For the weekends there are some terrific
brunch dishes in the recipe section, which take a bit longer
to cook and are more caloric, but because you will be eating just two meals on those days, you can get away with it.
There is the added advantage that you will have fasted for
about fourteen hours overnight.

What's so good about nuts?

Nuts have traditionally had a bad rap because they are oily
and high in calories. However, you will find some nuts in
the recipes because they are high in protein and fiber, they
are satiating, and they do not cause much upsurge in blood

that losing weight and maintaining an
significantly reduce your risk of prog
tes to diabetes. In a trial run by the
Health that recruited more than three
prediabetes, they found that a 7 pe
bined with an exercise regime cut
developing diabetes by 58 percent ov
For more on the Diabetes Preventi
.cdc.gov/diabetes/prevention/abou

Diet Timeline: W
and What to

The First Two

Once you've started, you will fi
weight fast. Some of it will be fat
be passing a lot of urine. It is esse
two to three quarts of calorie-f
become constipated and get hea
up to you, as long as it doesn't
ordinary tap water. If you are n
try disguising it by adding a s
fresh mint and cucumber. I lo
lemon, fruit-flavored tea, and
only a splash of milk). Some p
oddly enough, there is eviden
hunger. Drink zero-calorie so
juice and smoothies.

The first two weeks are likely to be the toughest, as your body adapts to fewer calories, but this should in turn lead to some dramatic changes. To give you a flavor of what you are likely to experience and the sort of changes you can expect I asked a friend of mine, Dick, who was about to start the diet, to keep a detailed diary.

"It Was How to Eat Less—but Eat Better"

Dick is a foodie. Nothing wrong with that, but he was eating big portions and drinking too much. "I am not a binge drinker," he told me, "but six o'clock used to be time for the first gin and tonic. And I don't mean a small one. Then most of a bottle of wine. Followed by a few whiskies." Dick may have been exaggerating—but only a little.

Even his nonalcoholic drinks were caloric. He would start each day with four sugars in his mug of tea.

At 215 pounds and with a 42-inch waist, he was overweight. He was beginning to look not only paunchy but also uncharacteristically gray and ill. Shortly after being diagnosed as a diabetic he contacted me for advice. We agreed that he would aim to lose 30 pounds (around 15 percent of his body weight) and get his blood sugars (which were over 163 mg/dl) back down to normal within eight weeks. He also wanted to lose 6 inches from his waist. He had a good-natured bet with his doctor, who said he wouldn't do it.

Over the first few weeks he managed not only to surprise his doctor but to disprove every cliché about rapid weight loss.

He didn't feel deprived. On Day 3 of the diet he wrote in his diary, "Still feeling fine. Weird. Not light-headed weird. Weird as in 'Everyone told me this wouldn't be possible and I'd be desperate enough to eat the dog, but that is so not the case.' "

By then his fasting glucose was already down 30 percent, and when he stood on the scale he found that he had lost 7 pounds in three days. As he wrote, "I know this will slow down but it's very motivating."

He did the cooking for himself and his wife, Alison. His meals were delicious: sea bass fillet with leafy greens, lemon sole with vegetables, baked chicken with red peppers, tomatoes, and onion. He put aside the bread, pasta, and potatoes.

He set himself a challenge: "The goal wasn't to worry about how I can survive on only 800 calories. It was 'How can I make those 800 calories really tasty and fulfilling?' It was how to eat less—but eat better."

After seven days, he had lost almost 10 pounds. By Day 9 his blood sugar levels had fallen to normal. His delight is clear in his diary: "Yes!! First result under the diabetes threshold!! For today I am not diabetic."

Two days later the reading was down again. He wrote: "Hello pancreas!"

He was hugely encouraged by the fact that it was all happening so rapidly. "You are dropping so fast. And it happens almost immediately." The fact that he was in control, doing something about his health, also spurred him on. "Just recently, life hadn't been the success it has always been in the past," he told me. "This turned that feeling around for me."

He maintained his work life and his social life. He kept on track by telling people what he was doing, avoiding refined carbohydrates, planning ahead, making sensible food choices. Dick would be the first to agree that it wasn't rocket science.

to blood sugar. You will find recipes here that include oats or brown rice—but in small quantities. It's a taste, not the main component of the meal. These carbohydrates are the slow-burning kind; they take time and energy to digest, which means you'll feel less hungry.

So what's going to keep me feeling full?

Fat and protein keep you feeling fuller for longer. The standard recommendations for protein are around 45 grams a day for a woman and 55 grams per day for a man. Good proteins to eat include eggs, fish, chicken, pork, shrimp, and tofu. Nuts, seeds, and legumes are packed full of protein too.

Is this a low-fat diet?

No—because, as I explained earlier, fat isn't the bad guy that it was once made out to be. It includes plenty of oily fish, a judicious amount of animal fat from meat, and plenty of plant fat (from nuts, seeds, olive oil, and avocados), as well as the fat in unsweetened yogurt. On the other hand, to lose weight fast you have to cut down on calories, so you won't find large amounts of cheese in the recipes.

Is snacking on fruit okay?

Fruit contains far more sugar than vegetables. There is some fruit in this diet, but it is rationed and used as an ingredient rather than an excuse to eat between meals. If you're looking for something to stir into yogurt, go for deep-colored blueberries, blackberries, cherries, or strawberries. But limit your intake of tropical fruit, which tends to be higher in sugar. And steer clear of dates and other dried fruit—eating two dates has the same effect on your blood sugar as eating two large basketfuls of strawberries.

Are some vegetables better than others?

Absolutely. Vegetables contain much less sugar than fruit, but some are starchier than others, which means they will affect your blood sugar. Leafy green vegetables such as spinach, cabbage, lettuce, kale, and chard are rich in vitamin C and fiber and very low in sugar and starch, as are broccoli and cauliflower, so dig in. Ditto for tomatoes, cucumbers, and peppers. It gets more complicated with root vegetables such as potatoes, parsnips, and turnips; these are quite high in starch, so they should be treated with more caution.

Do I have to eat breakfast?

It's a myth that everyone has to eat breakfast. I love it, but some people don't. For the weekends there are some terrific brunch dishes in the recipe section, which take a bit longer to cook and are more caloric, but because you will be eating just two meals on those days, you can get away with it. There is the added advantage that you will have fasted for about fourteen hours overnight.

What's so good about nuts?

Nuts have traditionally had a bad rap because they are oily and high in calories. However, you will find some nuts in the recipes because they are high in protein and fiber, they are satiating, and they do not cause much upsurge in blood sugar levels. They are an important component of the Mediterranean diet.

What about seeds?

Seeds may be tiny, but they're packed with nutrients such as protein, fiber, iron, vitamins, and omega-3 fatty acids. Whether it's chia seeds or flax, pumpkin seeds or hemp, sprinkle them in your salads, use them to make green vegetables more interesting, or stir them into yogurt. They will help you to feel fuller for longer. What's not to like?

Can I drink alcohol?

When you are on the diet, preferably not. If you have to, then stick to small amounts of spirits. Alcohol is highly caloric. A pint of beer contains around 180 calories. Ditto a large glass of wine. Red wine is lower in sugar than white, but the calories still add up. Five glasses of wine a week comes to 900 calories, the same as four doughnuts. Alcohol will also promote fat storage and inflammation in the liver, increasing the insulin resistance that promotes weight gain and diabetes. A number of people I have talked to while researching this book can date their blood sugar problems back to consuming too much booze.

What if I'm a prediabetic, not yet a type 2?

If, after doing the tests, you have discovered that you are prediabetic and overweight rather than fully diabetic, then you could certainly try doing the diet until you've got your blood sugars back to normal levels. There is good evidence that losing weight and maintaining an exercise program will significantly reduce your risk of progressing from prediabetes to diabetes. In a trial run by the National Institutes of Health that recruited more than three thousand people with prediabetes, they found that a 7 percent weight loss combined with an exercise regime cut the participants' risk of developing diabetes by 58 percent over the next five years.[37] For more on the Diabetes Prevention Program, visit www .cdc.gov/diabetes/prevention/about.htm.

Diet Timeline: What to Do and What to Expect

The First Two Weeks

Once you've started, you will find that you begin to lose weight fast. Some of it will be fat, but initially you will also be passing a lot of urine. It is essential that you drink at least two to three quarts of calorie-free fluid a day or you will become constipated and get headaches. What you drink is up to you, as long as it doesn't contain calories. It could be ordinary tap water. If you are not thrilled with plain water, try disguising it by adding a squeeze of lemon or lime, or fresh mint and cucumber. I love seltzer with lots of ice and lemon, fruit-flavored tea, and the occasional coffee (with only a splash of milk). Some people like drinking hot water; oddly enough, there is evidence that heat alone can soothe hunger. Drink zero-calorie sodas if you must. But avoid fruit juice and smoothies.

The first two weeks are likely to be the toughest, as your body adapts to fewer calories, but this should in turn lead to some dramatic changes. To give you a flavor of what you are likely to experience and the sort of changes you can expect I asked a friend of mine, Dick, who was about to start the diet, to keep a detailed diary.

"It Was How to Eat Less—but Eat Better"

Dick is a foodie. Nothing wrong with that, but he was eating big portions and drinking too much. "I am not a binge drinker," he told me, "but six o'clock used to be time for the first gin and tonic. And I don't mean a small one. Then most of a bottle of wine. Followed by a few whiskies." Dick may have been exaggerating—but only a little.

Even his nonalcoholic drinks were caloric. He would start each day with four sugars in his mug of tea.

At 215 pounds and with a 42-inch waist, he was overweight. He was beginning to look not only paunchy but also uncharacteristically gray and ill. Shortly after being diagnosed as a diabetic he contacted me for advice. We agreed that he would aim to lose 30 pounds (around 15 percent of his body weight) and get his blood sugars (which were over 163 mg/dl) back down to normal within eight weeks. He also wanted to lose 6 inches from his waist. He had a good-natured bet with his doctor, who said he wouldn't do it.

Over the first few weeks he managed not only to surprise his doctor but to disprove every cliché about rapid weight loss.

He didn't feel deprived. On Day 3 of the diet he wrote in his diary, "Still feeling fine. Weird. Not light-headed weird. Weird as in 'Everyone told me this wouldn't be possible and I'd be desperate enough to eat the dog, but that is so not the case.' "

By then his fasting glucose was already down 30 percent, and when he stood on the scale he found that he had lost 7 pounds in three days. As he wrote, "I know this will slow down but it's very motivating."

He did the cooking for himself and his wife, Alison. His meals were delicious: sea bass fillet with leafy greens, lemon sole with vegetables, baked chicken with red peppers, tomatoes, and onion. He put aside the bread, pasta, and potatoes.

He set himself a challenge: "The goal wasn't to worry about how I can survive on only 800 calories. It was 'How can I make those 800 calories really tasty and fulfilling?' It was how to eat less—but eat better."

After seven days, he had lost almost 10 pounds. By Day 9 his blood sugar levels had fallen to normal. His delight is clear in his diary: "Yes!! First result under the diabetes threshold!! For today I am not diabetic."

Two days later the reading was down again. He wrote: "Hello pancreas!"

He was hugely encouraged by the fact that it was all happening so rapidly. "You are dropping so fast. And it happens almost immediately." The fact that he was in control, doing something about his health, also spurred him on. "Just recently, life hadn't been the success it has always been in the past," he told me. "This turned that feeling around for me."

He maintained his work life and his social life. He kept on track by telling people what he was doing, avoiding refined carbohydrates, planning ahead, making sensible food choices. Dick would be the first to agree that it wasn't rocket science.

He started to walk more. Not just by going for actual walks but also by playing several rounds of golf a week. This added up to around four thousand extra steps a day.

The hunger wasn't hard to deal with, he found. Dick used the MyFitnessPal app, which scanned and measured everything he ate (and produced a report of calories and food contents) and took some of the emotion out of what he was eating—or, rather, not eating. He realized that the times when he thought he was hungry, it was often merely a craving, and if he did something else—walk the dog, for instance—the feeling would pass. Not being able to drink alcohol was admittedly trickier. After the first week he began to sneak in the odd whiskey. He still lost weight.

It wasn't all smooth sailing. There were days when his sugar levels nudged upward, but he didn't let these derail him. They were lapses, not relapses. The following day—helped by keeping the diary, which kept him mindful of why he was doing this—he got back on track.

It took Dick thirty-four days to see his blood sugar results stabilize in the normal range and two months to get down to 186 pounds. That was a year ago, and he maintains his weight loss by continuing to be active and eating low-carb. I haven't seen him looking so well for a long time. Occasionally he indulges in bread, but only a single slice, or he'll have a small portion of sweet potatoes. When he does this he sees his blood sugar levels rise, so he's decided it's simply not worth doing it that often.

The reasons he succeeded:

1. He was motivated.
2. He really believed the theory behind this rapid diet. It made sense to him.

3. He takes great pleasure in proving people wrong, especially his doctor—who hasn't yet paid up on their bet.
4. His wife, Alison, is a huge support.

After the First Two Weeks: Time to Review

Dick managed to lose 15 pounds in his first two weeks on the diet, and as his weight dropped, his blood sugar levels also fell. But though he had lost fat from his liver, his pancreas was still clogged. It was important he keep going, lose more inches around his waist. If he had stopped the diet at two weeks, his blood sugars probably would have gone back up again.

Not everyone needs to do the full eight weeks. If you are a prediabetic or slim to begin with (see Richard's story, below), then two weeks may be long enough for you to reach your goal—in which case you can move on to the Blood Sugar Way of Life (page 132).

Most overweight diabetics, however, will probably need to press on. Ideally you will have been not only doing the weight loss regime but also boosting your activity and mindfulness (see Chapters Eight and Nine). The important thing is how you are feeling, how you are coping. Here are a few questions to ask yourself:

1. Are you losing weight at a steady pace? By the end of the second week weight loss may have slowed, but it should still be rapid.

2. Is your appetite under better control? Most people report feeling less hungry by the end of the second week.

3. Are your blood sugar levels coming down or are they still all over the place?

4. Are you sleeping? If not, you may wish to eat your main meal a bit later.

5. Are you getting constipated? If so, I would recommend not only drinking more fluids but also adding more fiber-rich food—that is, nonstarchy vegetables.

6. Are you coping emotionally? You may feel more irritable, but what I would find more concerning would be a prolonged drop in mood.

7. Are you managing to stick with the diet most of the time?

If you answered no to more than two of these questions, then this may not be the right diet for you. Rather than give up, try what I call the 5:2 approach, where you cut your calories down to 800 for two days, staying on a low-carb Mediterranean-style eating plan for the rest of the week. It will be slower, but as long as you lose the weight it should still be effective. Details are on page 138.

The reason for doing a review at two weeks is that by now you should be in the swing of things, feeling in control, slimmer, and energized. But I also want to be sure that you are not pushing yourself too hard. Diets can be tough even if you are in perfect health. If you are a diabetic, there are added pitfalls.

I was recently contacted by John, who is in his early fifties. John has always been really fit and active. Earlier this year he began to feel tired and very thirsty all the time. So he went to his doctor, had a blood test, and discovered that his blood sugars were sky-high. His doctor thought, largely because of his age, that John must be a type 2 diabetic. Yet he was slim and a DEXA scan showed he had hardly any visceral fat. Nonetheless, John wanted to see if a very low-calorie diet would help. It didn't—after two weeks he had lost weight, but he didn't feel good and his blood sugars were still out of control, even on medication. He went back to his doctor, who decided he was probably not a type 2 after all but a late-onset type 1 diabetic.

Most type 1 diabetics develop the condition as children or in early adulthood, but some do so much later in life. John's blood sugar problems were caused not by too much liver fat but by damage his pancreas had suffered from his own immune system. He is now managing his blood sugar levels with medication and a relatively low-carb diet.

So John's story is a cautionary tale. Richard, on the other hand, is an example of just how effective rapid weight loss can be if your problem really is too much visceral fat.

"At Work They Started Calling Me the 'Disappearing Man'"

We all have different personal fat thresholds, and there can be quite wide variations between the points at which people start to see big improvements in their blood sugar control. Richard Doughty managed to get his blood sugar under control in eleven days—less time than an average family's summer vacation.

How did the fifty-nine-year-old journalist do it? "It was such a shock, getting the diagnosis," he says. "But I can be very single-minded." He chose a time when his wife was away—"I didn't want her to worry. And she might think that I was being a bit nuts"—and when he didn't have any big family events scheduled. He made sure he carried on his life in just the same way as before—he went to work and continued to play sports.

For Richard, one of the hardest things about the diet was being told he looked too thin! Because Doughty is one of those skinny-fat people I mentioned earlier, a TOFI—no one was more surprised than he to discover his blood sugar status. When he started losing weight people told him he was too scrawny. "At work they started calling me the 'disappearing man,'" he says. "But better to look too thin than to be missing a foot."

He lost 9 pounds in eleven weeks—by which time his blood sugars had returned to normal. He waited two months before he saw his doctor again, and when he did go back for another check, his blood sugar levels were still comfortably below the diabetes mark. He has since had regular tests and each time the results are fine. When he talks about the turnaround you can still hear the delight in his voice. He dieted his way back to health in less time than it takes for a tennis player to win Wimbledon.

The Four-Week Review

The next key moment in your dieting odyssey will be the four-week review. By now you will be halfway through the diet, and hopefully things are going well. You will have lost a lot of weight, with much of it coming off your waist. Your blood sugars will be starting to stabilize at close to normal levels. Your sugar cravings will likely be much reduced.

Retake our "Do You Crave Carbs?" quiz on page 69 and see how you are doing. And ideally you should revisit your doctor to repeat blood tests and scans, if you've previously done them.

Just as with the two-week review, by the end of four weeks some will have reached their goals, in which case they should celebrate and move on to the maintenance phase (see page 126). Others may be finding it hard going, but if that's you, don't give up—moving to a 5:2 approach or going straight to the maintenance program are viable options.

So, what changes can you realistically expect to see in your weight and blood sugars by the end of four weeks? Well, in Dr. Taylor's original study, his volunteers, who started out at over 200 pounds, had lost an average of 22 pounds by the end of four weeks, most of it fat.[38] They had also lost nearly 3 inches from their waist. Other changes that happened by four weeks included:

Fasting glucose	Down from 166 to 103 mg/dl
Fasting insulin	Down from 151 to 57 pmol/l
GGT (liver test)	Down from 62 to 25 U/1

As I mentioned earlier, however, when Dr. Taylor did a second study with people who were older and had been diabetic for much longer, the results were mixed.[39] Those who had been diabetic for less than four years did really well. But those who'd been diabetic for more than eight years and were on lots of medication were less likely to see rapid improvements in their blood sugar levels.

That said, everyone reported feeling better, sleeping better, and being more active. Blood pressure and cholesterol levels also improved across the board.

At the End of Eight Weeks

By the end of the eight-week diet, if not before, you will see some big changes in your body shape and biochemistry. You should be sleeping better and feeling a real sense of achievement. Perhaps you need to buy some new clothes to fit your new, slimmer self; maybe you stop and look in mirrors to admire the difference. So pull out that old photo. Take a new one. Post them on Facebook or Twitter.

By the end of eight weeks most people will have reached their targets, but some won't. Perhaps you have more weight to lose; maybe your blood sugar or A1C results have not improved as much as you'd hoped for. If you feel you are heading in the right direction but are just not quite there yet, I suggest that rather than continue eating 800 calories every day, you move to the more flexible 5:2 approach (see page 138).

The end of the diet is also a good time to visit your doctor, redo the tests, and celebrate what you have done with family and friends.

Getting this far is a real achievement, but you don't want to undo all the good work by going back to living the way you used to. Your main preoccupation now should be, "How am I going to stay in this shape for the rest of my life?"

The Blood Sugar Way of Life

As I'm sure you know, many people who go on a diet end up gaining back some, if not most, of the weight they have so painfully lost. But this is not inevitable. The main thing you have to do is create a lifestyle you can stick to. If this involves avoiding all your favorite foods and running twenty miles a day, then it will fail. Be realistic.

Don't despair. Lots of others have lost weight and kept it off. I lost 20 pounds three years ago, and occasionally I put a couple of pounds back on. But I find I can rapidly lose them again. I'm sure the main reason I've succeeded in keeping off the weight is because I've gone from gorging on sugary carbs to following a Mediterranean-style eating plan. That, along with increased activity and practicing mindfulness (see Chapter Nine), has helped me keep diabetes at bay.

The following are a few other things I've found useful and which are now a way of life for me. They are based on numerous conversations with diet experts.

- Try to sit down at the kitchen table for every meal. If you eat on the run or in front of the TV, you will eat badly and go on eating well beyond the point that you would normally feel full. A striking example of this was when researchers from the University of Southern California gave people going into a movie theater buckets of stale popcorn.[40] The people who normally eat popcorn at the movies wolfed it down, despite the fact it tasted terrible. This demonstrates how little attention we pay to what we are eating when we are distracted.

- Try to eat slowly. It takes time for the food you eat to reach the parts of your small intestine where cells release a hormone, PYY, that tells your brain, *I'm full.* That's why you will eat less if you eat slowly. During a meal, I regularly put my knife and fork down for a while and try to wait half a minute or so before picking them up again. I also now leave food on my plate when I am no longer hungry, even though that goes against everything I was taught when I was growing up.

- Avoid "diet" products. Typically, diet products are highly processed and often contain sugar and/ or sweeteners (which may not switch off hunger signals).

- Eat a lot of soup. It is filling, cheap, and practical. We make big quantities, often out of leftover vegetables, and freeze what we don't eat right away, so there's always some ready to be defrosted and heated up.

- Don't drink lots of alcohol. Alcohol contains plenty of calories and makes you disinhibited, so you are more likely to snack. I have switched to drinking red wine and try to drink only when I am eating. I also leave the bottle on the other side of the room because I know that I am less likely to fill my glass regularly if I have to get up. For similar reasons we leave the salt in the cupboard rather than on the table, and the food gets left on the stovetop rather than put on the table. I am less likely to help myself to more if I have to cross the room.

- Keep tempting foods out of the house or out of sight. The kids sometimes sneak chocolate and cookies in, but they know better than to leave them anywhere I can find them. In a fascinating study Cornell University researchers went around to houses in Syracuse, New York, taking photos of people's kitchens. They found they could predict a family's weight by the foods left out and visible. If breakfast cereals, for example, were visible, then the owners were on average 21 pounds heavier than people in households where the cereals were tucked away. Breakfast cereals have a reputation for being healthful, but generally they aren't.[41]

- Keep your cupboards well stocked. If there's no food in the house, then you will probably wind up getting take-out. Make sure there's plenty of healthful food around, such as nuts, yogurt, and eggs. Keep the fridge stocked with carrot sticks, green peppers, or tomatoes, perhaps with some salsa or hummus, for moments when you just have to snack. Put them at eye level in the fridge. Anything too high in calories needs to be covered up and put at the bottom of the fridge where you are less likely to see it.

- Know your weaknesses. Mine is toast, and I did suggest to my wife we throw the toaster out (on the grounds I would rarely bother to use the grill), but she refused. Instead I keep unsalted nuts by the toaster, so when I am tempted to snack on toast and jam, I eat nuts instead. (Mostly.)

- Weigh yourself several times a week. Scales can be extraordinary fickle; sometimes my weight seems to go up and down like a yo-yo. There is a widely held belief that you shouldn't weigh yourself more than once a week. Yet a recent study suggests more is better. In this particular trial, researchers followed forty people attending a health promotion program.[42] Some weighed themselves daily, others weekly, monthly, or hardly at all. The more often people weighed themselves, the more weight they lost.

- Wear a belt. One of the surest ways of telling that you are putting on unhealthy fat is when your belt starts to feel tight again.

- Take extra care when you go out for a meal. When we're dining out, I make sure the server never leaves the bread basket on the table, or I would just help myself. I stick to one course, with lots of vegetables instead of rice or potatoes. I rarely have dessert, and when I do, I always share it with someone else. Research shows that eating a small amount of something sweet, sticky, and tasty is just as satisfying as eating a large amount.

- Try not to go grocery shopping on an empty stomach. I always eat *before* I go to the grocery store, as that way I'm less likely to buy high-carb, unhealthful foods on impulse. I aim to fill half the basket, at least, with healthful stuff. If I pick up a cake, I always look at the label—the huge number of calories and vast amounts of sugar normally make me put it back on the shelf. I used to kid myself that if I bought a whole cake or a package of cookies I would eat only a small amount, but now I realize that's not true. For the same reason I never buy large bars of chocolate, however much of a bargain they seem.

- Take the stairs. Instead of taking the elevator, I take the stairs—and normally I try to run up them. I think it is sad how many people stand in elevators or on escalators when they could be burning a few extra calories by walking up the steps.

- Have a strategy for handling cravings. When I get a craving for something sweet, I buy sugar-free chewing gum. Cravings are all about imagining the tastes and textures of the forbidden food. It is almost impossible to think about the taste of chocolate when you are munching on gum.

- Get a dog to walk. Our dog, Tari, barks loudly if we don't take her for a walk at least once a day. (Maybe not the most practical tip if you live in the city or prefer cats!)

- Keep busy. Take up a new hobby that will keep your body and mind active. I took up Latin dance—it got my heart going and was mentally challenging.

- Acknowledge three good things. This is based on an idea devised by psychologist Martin Seligman. At the end of the day, think of and/or write down three things that went well that day. It doesn't have to be much—perhaps someone complimented you, or you watched a beautiful sunset. The point is that it focuses your attention on the positive. It is a good way to lift your mood and bolster resilience.

- Try to fast each week. I have one day when I try to go at least twelve hours without food. I do this by having breakfast, skipping lunch, and having a light evening meal. There are health benefits from short periods of fasting; it also reminds me that I can control my hunger, and it does not control me.

What If I Can't Keep to 800 Calories Every Day?

The less intensive BSD—Going 5:2

We are all different. Many people—including those who have provided the case studies for this book—find 800 calories a day surprisingly easy and just keep going. It does work well for people who are motivated, and I hope that is how it works out for you.

But no one diet is going to suit everyone. If you begin the diet and really don't feel well on it, or if you find 800 calories a day every day either too tough or too inconvenient to stick to for the full eight weeks, then I would recommend the 5:2 approach as a gentler alternative.

The 5:2 approach is very simple. For five days of the week you don't count calories but instead simply stick to the low-carb Mediterranean diet I described earlier. Then, for two days a week, you cut down your calories to 800 a day using the menus in this book. You can do this on any two days of the week that suit you, but it is best to be consistent so that you get into a pattern. Try consecutive days, such as Monday and Tuesday. Or you may prefer to split your days, going Monday and Thursday. Do whatever works for you.

You won't lose weight as fast as you would if you stick to 800 calories a day, but it can be more effective than conventional dieting. Studies suggest the 5:2 approach is easier to stick to; you lose fat (rather than muscle) faster, and you see bigger improvements in your insulin sensitivity.[43]

I've written extensively about the health and weight loss benefits of the 5:2 "intermittent fasting" approach in *The FastDiet* (thefastdiet.co.uk). In the original version of *The FastDiet*, I recommended that men stick to 600 calories a day and women to 500 calories twice a week. Going up to 800 calories is unlikely to make that much of a difference, particularly if you are low-carb on the other five days.

The 5:2 diet was how I reversed my own diabetes, and since I wrote that book I have had many emails from former diabetics, including one from Leo, who had been a type 2 diabetic for twelve years. Despite being on medication, Leo found that his blood sugars were getting so bad that in 2012 his doctor told him he needed to start on insulin injections. Instead Leo did my 5:2 diet, lost 44 pounds in three months, and was able to stop all his diabetes medication. Three years later he has put on a few pounds, but his blood sugars remain fine.

What Should I Do About Checkups?

If you were prediabetic and you have a personal blood glucose monitor, then I would recommend, at least initially, that you do monthly fasting blood sugar checks after you finish the eight weeks, just to make sure you are keeping on track. You also need to have yearly blood sugar checks by your doctor, at least initially. If you go back to your previous lifestyle and activity levels, then over time you are at risk of becoming prediabetic again.

If you were a type 2 diabetic, then you will need to go on having regular checkups with your doctor. Usually this will be at least yearly. If your blood sugar levels remain in the normal range, then your doctor may be happy to arrange these checks less often. But don't just stop going, as it is important to make sure your kidneys, eyes, cardiovascular system, feet, and other organs have not been affected.

What Should I Do If Things Start Going in the Wrong Direction?

First of all, review your diet. Are you slipping in more of the high-GI simple carbohydrates than you need? Have your portions gotten bigger? If you are serious about wanting to stay healthy, then you will have to act. This may involve simply cutting out the extra treats you have allowed yourself, or adding in a few weeks of intermittent fasting (see the 5:2 option above). Some people make the 5:2 approach their maintenance program, or they go for a 6:1 approach (having one day a week when they stick to 800 calories). Research shows that you can get metabolic benefits, such as improved insulin sensitivity, from fasting even just one day a week.

Next, review your exercise and activity levels. Are you still taking the stairs, a regular walk, and fitting in some resistance exercises (see Chapter Eight)?

Are you going through a period of disruption and stress in your life? If so, the increased cortisol levels can upset your blood sugars. Chapter Nine is all about techniques to de-stress and reduce the need for comfort eating.

Finally, don't despair or give up. Putting on a bit of weight after you have stopped dieting is normal, so don't blame or chastise yourself. The main thing is to get back on track as swiftly as possible. This book offers science-based guidelines and lots of specific advice, but the important thing is that you fine-tune that advice so it works for you. Joining an online community of like-minded souls can be very helpful for getting helpful advice or simply sharing experiences.

CHAPTER EIGHT

Getting Active

EXERCISE IS HUGELY IMPORTANT FOR HEALTH, PARticularly if you have difficulty controlling your blood sugar levels. As we have seen, the starting point for most type 2 diabetes is insulin resistance, a condition in which your body stops responding to insulin, forcing your pancreas to produce ever larger amounts of it. And the quickest and most effective way to reduce insulin resistance is to do more exercise.[44]

The problem is that many people find doing exercise tedious or unpleasant. In this chapter I present a program that will give you the maximum benefit in the minimum time.

The Simplest of Simple Starts

The first and easiest thing you can do is stand every thirty minutes. You should start doing this right from week one of the diet. Try putting this book down and doing it right now.

The evidence that sitting kills goes back to the 1950s, when a study was done comparing bus conductors (who stand) with bus drivers (who sit). It turned out that the bus drivers had twice the risk of developing heart disease as the conductors.[45]

Since then we have become a lot more sedentary. We sit at work, in the car, and at home, moving only to shift from one seat to another. Many of us spend more than half our waking lives, at least eight hours a day, sitting on our bottoms looking at computers or watching television.

The effects of this on our bodies are dire. One of the largest studies ever carried out, involving nearly 800,000 people, found that those who are sedentary have:[46]

- Twice the chance of developing type 2 diabetes
- Twice the chance of dying from a heart attack or stroke

Another way of putting this is that every hour you spend sitting down doing something like watching television cuts about twenty minutes off your life.[47]

It's not just the time spent sitting that matters but time spent sitting continuously. In a recent study from Australia, researchers gathered seventy healthy adults and asked them to sit for nine hours.[48] Every few hours they had to eat, and their blood sugar and insulin levels were measured. Then they did it all over again, except this time they got up every thirty minutes and walked around for a bit. Just by standing up and walking every thirty minutes they reduced their blood sugar levels by 39 percent and their insulin levels by 26 percent.

So get an app with an alarm that will remind you to move every thirty minutes. If you watch a lot of TV, set a timer and go for a quick stroll during the commercial breaks. You could set an alarm that goes off in another room, so that you have to get up to go turn it off. Or keep the remote control beside the TV instead of next to you, so you have to get up to change channels. Television is designed to hook you in (I should know, I work in it), and the only way to combat its insidious charms is to be aware of its dangers.

Take a Stand

If you are sitting less, you are likely to be standing more. Many famous thinkers, including Leonardo da Vinci and Ernest Hemingway, found that they did their best work while standing.

But is it practical? And how much difference would it make if we stood more? To find out, I watched Dr. John Buckley and a team of researchers from the University of Chester as they conducted a simple experiment.[49] They asked ten people who work in an office to try standing for at least three hours a day for one week. Their normal desks were put away and replaced by special standing desks.

All the volunteers were equipped with accelerometers (movement monitors) to record just how much moving around they were doing. They also wore glucose monitors that measured their blood sugar levels constantly, day and night.

Some of the volunteers were nervous beforehand, saying things like, "I think my feet might hurt," "My back won't be able to stand it," or "I've never stood for as long as three hours." But in fact, they all stuck with it.

What effects did it have on their bodies? Well, the first thing we discovered is that the volunteers had much better control of their blood sugar. After they ate a meal, their blood sugar levels fell back to normal far more quickly than before. They also burned an extra 50 calories an hour. If you stand for three hours a day for five days a week, that's around 750 calories a week. Over the course of a year it would add up to 30,000 extra calories, or around 8 pounds of fat. "That's the equivalent of running about ten marathons a year," Dr. Buckley says, "just by standing up three or four hours in your day." And one woman with arthritis found that standing actually improved her symptoms.

We can't all stand up at work, but even small adjustments, such as standing while talking on the phone and going over to talk to a colleague rather than sending an email, will help.

Walk the Walk

Even better than standing is walking. Walking is the great elixir of life, and you should aim to do 10,000 steps a day.

This is the minimum that is recommended to keep you healthy and help keep weight off.

In Chapter Six, in the "Before You Start" section, I asked you to record how many steps you take over a typical week, so that you can monitor any increase. You won't want to go from zero to 100 mph, so aim for a steady build. Most people average around 5,000 steps a day (those who are older and overweight tend to do less). If you increase the number of steps you do a day by 500 for every week you are on the Blood Sugar Diet, you should be close to the magic 10,000 number by the end of eight weeks.

In other words, if you normally do 5,000 steps a day, then at the start of week one you should aim to do 5,500 steps a day. During week two it'll be 6,000 steps a day, and so on. You will find that as you lose weight you will become more energized and feel more willing to be active.

As you are going to be walking more, you should invest in comfortable shoes. You may even want to buy special walking socks with extra padding.

So how are you going to boost the number of steps you take? Ideally you will do it by building it into your day so that it is not a chore, just something you do without thinking.

My personal rules are:

1. I always take the stairs. I work on the seventh floor of a building in central London, and it is 200 steps up and down. I do that at least twice a day. That comes to 800 steps.

2. I always walk or run on escalators.

3. When I am traveling around central London I always walk, if the journey is less than a mile, or I bike if it is longer. I have a fold-up bike that I have spray-painted bright green so it is less likely to get stolen, and I take this to work with me most days.

4. I live a mile from our local train station, up a steep hill. I always bike or walk to and from the station. Walking a mile is about 2,000 steps.

Other ways to build more steps into your life include:

- Take public transport. Get off the bus one stop earlier.

- Listen to upbeat music or an audio book—it can make walking more pleasurable.

- Leave your car at the far end of the parking lot when you go to the mall or supermarket.

- When you are at an airport, walk around rather than just sitting there killing time. Walking before a flight helps with jet lag, too.

- When you are at work, pace around between meetings. Go and see colleagues in person rather than send emails. Stand while you are on the phone (research suggests this will also make you sound more assertive than when you are sitting).

- You might consider buying a treadmill desk. It allows you to walk while working at your desk. It is not something I have ever attempted, but here's a link to a report by a BBC journalist who did give it a try: www.bbc.co.uk/news/magazine-21076461.

- Take up activities like gardening, painting, or dancing, which require more movement.

- When you are on vacation, join a guided walking tour. These group tours normally last one to two hours, are very cheap and sometimes even free, and are led by knowledgeable, personable guides. I've so far done this in Dublin, Berlin, London, Sydney, and Paris. My kids, who really don't enjoy walking, are now very enthusiastic about these tours.

- Join a walking group or form your own. I have friends from Australia, Tim and Clare, and every year we aim to spend three or four days doing part of a classic English walk, such as the coast-to-coast (you walk from one side of England to the other). We do ten to twelve miles a day and make a long weekend of it.

Tip: *If you want to get maximum bang for your buck, then it is better to throw in a bit of fast walking rather than simply going for a gentle amble.*

In a Danish study, thirty-two diabetics were asked either to walk at a moderate pace for five hours a week or to alternate three minutes of walking fast with three minutes of walking slow, again for five hours a week.[50] After four months the group doing the fast-slow regime had lost an average of 6.6 pounds.

Strength Training

Up until you're thirty, your muscles get bigger. Then, if you don't use them, they get smaller. You can lose 5 percent of your muscle mass every decade from age thirty onward.

To keep your muscles, you have to do some form of resistance training. You could go to the gym, or try what I do, which is a simple regime designed to be done anytime, anyplace, anywhere. With my plan you exercise as many major muscle groups as possible, and alternate between them, so the ones not being worked get a bit of a rest. I start with push-ups (working the upper body), then follow these with something that works the core (abdominal crunches) or the legs (squats).

What I do is based on a paper in the American College of Sports Medicine's *Health and Fitness Journal*, and I do it at least three times a week, first thing in the morning.[51] It only takes a few minutes. My favorite exercises are push-ups, squats, abdominal crunches, the biceps curl, and the plank.

> **Push-ups.** Get into a push-up position with the palms
> of your hands under your shoulders and the balls
> of your feet touching the ground. Keep your body

straight. Lower your body till your elbows form a 90-degree angle and then push up. If you find this too hard, do it with your knees on the ground.

Squats. Stand with feet apart. Bend from the hips, keeping your weight on your heels. Make sure your back is straight. Keep bending until the legs are at a 90-degree angle—imagine you are preparing to sit in a chair. Push back up without bending your back. Squats work the biggest muscles in your body. If you want to make this harder, add weights.

Crunches. Lie on your back with knees bent, feet flat on the floor, and your hands by the side of your head. Curl up your upper body without lifting your lower back off the floor. Make sure your chin is tucked in toward your chest. When your shoulders and upper back are lifted off the floor, curl back down.

Biceps curls. This requires a small handheld weight. Stand with feet apart and hands by your side, with one hand clutching the small weight. Then, with your arm kept by your side, raise your hand by bending your elbow. Transfer the weight to your other hand and repeat.

Plank. Lie on the floor and then raise yourself onto your forearms and toes so that your body forms a straight line from head to toe. Make sure your midsection doesn't rise or drop. Squeeze your buttocks and hold the position for as long as possible. Remember, this position should never cause pain in the lower back.

I suggest you start in week one of the diet by doing one set of 10 repetitions of each of these (with 20-second holds on the planks): 10 push-ups, 10 squats, 10 crunches, 10 biceps curls, and 10 planks. Do this three times in the first week. Aim for two sets of 10 repetitions in the second week, and three sets by the fourth week.

Getting More Vigorous Activity

The standard recommendations are to do at least 150 minutes of moderate aerobic activity (walking, swimming, mowing the lawn) or 75 minutes of vigorous aerobic activity (running, cycling, dancing) a week. Most of us don't get close.

That's why I like HIT (high-intensity training), a completely different approach. It is short but intense. I do it at home, but it is best, at least to start with, if it is done in a supervised setting such as a gym. As with any other form of exercise, it would be wise to discuss it with your doctor before starting, particularly if you are on medication.

High-Intensity Training (HIT)

I was introduced to this form of exercise four years ago by Dr. Jamie Timmons of Kings College, London. When I first met him he shocked me by saying that I could get most of the more important benefits of exercise from doing just three minutes a week of intensive cycling. I thought this sounded too good to be true, but I'm always up for a challenge, so I decided to give it a try.

Before I started they did some blood work and measured my fasting insulin and glucose. Then for the next six weeks I got on my exercise bike three times a week and pedaled away, following a regime that Dr. Timmons recommended (see box on pages 154–55). It was quite tough to start with, but I soon got used to it. My family also got used to the strange grunting noises I made as I pushed myself as hard as I could.

At the end of six weeks I went back to Dr. Timmons's lab, had my blood work done again, and discovered that my insulin sensitivity had improved by an impressive 24 percent, which is broadly in line with what they expected (some will improve more, others less).

So how does it work?

According to Jamie, if you are doing something very active, like HIT, you are breaking down the body's stores of glucose, deposited in your muscles as glycogen. Smash up these glycogen stores and you create room for more sugar to be sucked out of your blood after a meal.

Compared with standard exercise regimes, people who do HIT see a bigger loss in abdominal fat, which, as we've seen, is important because abdominal fat is so closely tied to the risk of developing diabetes and heart disease.

Michael's HIT Regime

My regime consists of three bursts of twenty seconds, done three times a week on an exercise bike. You should attempt this only once you have built up some fitness. If you are out of shape, you should start by doing the beginner's regime I describe in the next section.

1. Get on an exercise bike and do a short warm-up of gentle cycling against limited resistance. You should just about notice the effort in your thighs.

2. After a couple of minutes, begin pedaling fast, then swiftly crank up the resistance. The amount of resistance you select will depend on your strength and fitness. It should be high enough that after fifteen seconds of sprinting you can feel it. If after fifteen seconds you can still keep going at the same pace

A Slow-Build Regime for Beginners

I like doing the three blasts of twenty seconds, but unless you are already quite fit you should start with something that is less demanding. The following is suggested for type 2 diabetics and those who are not particularly fit.

Week one: Pedal on an exercise bike for a few minutes. When you feel ready, crank up the speed and pedal hard against resistance for ten seconds. When without too much effort, then the resistance you've chosen isn't high enough. It mustn't, however, be so high that you grind to a complete halt. It's a matter of experimenting. What you'll find is that as you get fitter, the amount of resistance you can cope with increases. It's not speed but effort you are after.

3. After your first burst of fast sprinting, drop the resistance and do a couple of minutes of gentle pedaling to get your breath back.

4. Then repeat the bursts twice more, with a couple of minutes of gentle pedaling in between.

5. Finish with a couple of minutes of gentle cycling to allow your heart rate and blood pressure to return to normal before stepping off the bike.

In total it takes me less than ten minutes.

you catch your breath and go back to pedaling slowly until you've been on the bike for a total of ten minutes. Do this three times in week one.

Week two: Do the same thing as in week one, but this time you fit two 10-second bursts into your ten-minute ride. Separate the bursts with a couple of minutes of gentle cycling, giving you time to recover.

Weeks three and four: By now you should be able to manage to push your short bursts up to fifteen seconds.

So you will be doing two bursts of fifteen seconds within a ten-minute cycle ride, and you will be doing this three times a week

Weeks five and six: Try to do two 20-second bursts in your ten-minute ride. You may be tempted to go on for longer than twenty seconds. Don't. Going for longer won't make it better and may make it worse.

Weeks seven onward: You can stick to two 20-second bursts, or you can try moving on to three 20-second bursts. Just be sure that you are not pushing yourself too hard.

Summary

Stand up every thirty minutes.

Starting from your current level, add an extra 500 steps a day each week, until you reach 10,000 steps a day.

Do strength exercises three times a week. Begin slowly and add in more reps each week.

If you want to try HIT, it's best to start in a gym, where you will be properly supervised.

You can get a more detailed program in my book *FastExercise*, or download the FastExercise app.

CHAPTER NINE

Sorting Out Your Head

S TRESS AND BLOOD SUGAR PROBLEMS ARE VERY strongly linked. High levels of the stress hormone cortisol make your muscles and other tissues more insulin-resistant. Stress reduces insulin's ability to get sugar into cells. Stress hormones also stimulate your liver to release more sugar into your blood. Furthermore, stress is an important cause of insomnia and weight gain. When you feel stressed, you are far more likely to give in to carb cravings and comfort eating.

To keep weight off permanently, you need to change the way you think about food and deal with setbacks. Many people who get their blood sugar back under control are changed by the experience. Remember Carlos? He was so sick he thought he was about to die. Now he works with overeaters as a diabetes buddy. Geoff Whitington is also a diabetes champion—audiences love him because they can relate to his experiences. Bob Smietana, the Chicago journalist who regularly ate doughnuts for breakfast, is training to run marathons. All of them have sustained their weight loss by making it part of who they are and reminding themselves how far they have come.

Cassie, the nurse, put it powerfully when she wrote: "It is the best feeling in the world not having to take insulin anymore. Every time I'm tempted to eat something I shouldn't, I say to myself, 'If you eat that, then you will be back on insulin,' and the temptation goes. I have been in a food prison for so long: thinking about what I want to eat and then, when I've eaten it, feeling guilty about what I've just eaten. I don't do that anymore. I now think about life and living, and I get so much more done!"

That said, there are always going to be difficult and stressful days when things are going badly and you reach for a large container of ice cream or a family-sized bar of chocolate. If you give in (and most of us will at some time in our lives), then beware of a common dieting pitfall: catastrophic thinking.

Imagine that, for whatever reason, you have a bit of a splurge. Instead of thinking, "That was a one-time thing; I'm only human," you say to yourself, "I'm a weak-willed failure, I will never succeed, I'm never going to be able to stay off all sugar, I might as well give up now." The results of giving in to catastrophic thinking can be catastrophic gorging.

On TV I recently saw an experiment where a group of dieters were divided into two teams and then, separately, taken to a cake-making lesson. Just before they started, the members of Team A were offered a slice of cake. After they had eaten it they were told they had just eaten 750 calories. Those on Team B were offered a slice of the same cake, but they were told that the slice they had eaten was only 190 calories. Then both groups spent an afternoon making cakes while being secretly filmed.

Team A, who felt they had already blown their diet, decided, *What the hell,* and began eating any spare pieces of cake they could vacuum up. They ended up eating more than four pounds of cake between the four of them. Team B, who thought they'd only had a modest treat, were much more restrained, and though they ate some extra cake, it was far less.

The lesson is, watch out for tricky psychologists. But also watch out for catastrophic thinking. One way to counter this is to be aware you are doing it. Another way is to practice mindfulness.

Mindfulness: Reducing Stress

Many of us go through life with self-critical and unhelpful thoughts rattling around inside our heads, each thought competing for our attention. These constant mental meanderings can lead to a spiral of overeating, self-loathing, depression, and insomnia.

Saying "pull yourself together" rarely works. But you can counter these negative thoughts by making yourself more mindful. Instead of obsessing, take time out to look at yourself and your thoughts in a less judgmental, more reasonable way.

Mindfulness is a modern take on the ancient practice of meditation. The good news is that you don't need to be religious or retreat to a Tibetan monastery to do it. You can buy books about mindfulness, but it's not really something you need to read about; it's something you need to do. I recommend joining a group or downloading an app, such as Headspace, created by former monk Andy Puddicombe, which will guide you through the process.

With an app, the sessions are short: at first it's just ten minutes, then fifteen minutes, and finally twenty minutes. This is not a particularly time-consuming thing to do. You may be cynical, but it really is worth trying. I find it reduces cravings and helps me sleep better.

When I'm doing a mindfulness session I sit in a comfortable chair, turn on my app, rest my hands on my thighs, and close my eyes. Then, guided by the app, I spend the next few minutes trying to focus on my breath. I pay attention to the sensation of the breath going through my nostrils, filling my chest, expanding and contracting my diaphragm. I try to stay focused on this task; when I notice that my thoughts have drifted, which they do, I bring them back to the breath.

I try to treat thoughts like balloons that drift into my consciousness; once I have noticed they are there, I simply allow them to drift away. I say "simply," but when you first start you will find it's almost impossible to stop thinking about deadlines, food, the overdraft on your checking account, the kids, your ex-partner, and on and on. You might start wondering, "This isn't working. What is Michael Mosley raving about?" Put those suspicious thoughts aside; it will get easier. Like any skill, practice makes perfect.

Mindfulness can be very effective in a surprisingly short time. In a study published in the journal *Social Cognitive and Affective Neuroscience*, researchers took fifteen volunteers who had never tried anything like this and put them through a brain scanner.[52] They also got them to fill out an anxiety questionnaire. The volunteers then did four sessions of mindfulness training, spread over four days. Then the tests were repeated.

After the participants completed the mindfulness training, anxiety ratings fell by 39 percent. The scans also revealed increased activity in the areas of the brain that control worrying, particularly the ventromedial prefrontal cortex and the anterior cingulate gyrus. This supports the claim that mindfulness strengthens our ability to ignore negative thoughts and feelings.

To get a flavor of what mindfulness can do for you, try either or both of the following:

Breathing exercise. Go into a quiet room and sit with your eyes closed. Breathe in and out of your nose, slowly counting to four as you inhale and again to four as you exhale. Use very shallow breaths; don't let your chest rise and fall. Set a timer and do this for three minutes.

Progressive muscle relaxation. In the 1920s, Dr. Edmund Jacobson developed a system of tensing and totally relaxing specific muscle groups. A study published in the journal *Diabetes Care* showed that five weekly sessions of this kind of therapy helped

How to Do Progressive Muscle Relaxation

Sit in a chair with your feet flat on the floor. Close your eyes. When you tense a muscle, hold the tension for five seconds and then relax for thirty seconds before you go on to the next tensing movement. After you are done, breathe in deeply and stretch.

Right hand and forearm: Make a fist and then release.

Right upper arm: Bend the arm and make a muscle, then release.

Left hand and forearm: Make a fist and then release.

Left upper arm: Bend the arm to make a muscle, then release.

Forehead: Raise your eyebrows and then relax your face.

Eyes and cheeks: Squeeze the eyes and then relax.

Mouth and jaw: Clench your teeth and pull the corners of mouth down and relax.

to reduce blood sugar levels. It is easiest if someone guides you through this, rather than you trying to do it and read this book at the same time. Or you can just record your own voice instructing you what to do.

Shoulders and neck: Lock your hands behind your neck and push the back of the head against this resistance (don't move the head). Pull up your shoulders and press your head back against their resistance in a horizontal movement.

Chest and back: Breathe in deeply and hold your breath, pressing the shoulders together at the back at the same time, then let your shoulders hang and breathe normally.

Belly: Tighten the abs and then release.

Right thigh: Move the right foot forward against resistance and then release.

Right calf: Lift up the right heel and then relax.

Right foot: Bend the toes and then release.

Left thigh: Move the left foot forward against resistance and then release.

Left calf: Lift up the left heel and then relax.

Left foot: Bend the toes and then release.

Conclusion

So that's it. I know, it's quite a lot to digest. Elevated blood sugar is a serious threat, but I am greatly encouraged by research showing how we can combat and reverse it.

The link between high blood sugar and fat is clear. It's not so much the fat in your diet as the fat in your midriff—abdominal fat, visceral fat, the fat that infiltrates your liver and your pancreas. Get rid of that (or preferably stop it building up in the first place) and so many problems will go away.

There are lots of reasons why we are where we are, including the way that the food industry responded to the emphasis on low-fat diets by removing fat from their products and pumping them full of sugar instead. Now, however, there is evidence that the tide is turning, with consumers saying that added sugars are one of their biggest concerns.

But we also have to—collectively, as a society, I think—change the mind-set that says that it's okay to give ourselves and our children endless little treats. Snacking is not just a guilty pleasure; it's helping drive the diabesity epidemic.

If you've got type 2 diabetes, prediabetes, or just elevated blood sugar, then the message of this book is clear: *do something about it.* Don't assume that drugs will make it better or that your doctor has all the answers. If you've been wondering whether you might have blood sugar problems, or if you have a friend or relative you think might be at risk, then do get tested. The longer you ignore it, the worse things get.

Pharmaceutical companies are scrambling to develop new drugs. Surgeons are perfecting and promoting operations for weight loss. That is where a lot of research money is going. But I believe that many people, given the choice, would rather heal themselves through weight loss and diet. One of the things that has thrilled me most over the two years that I've been working on this book has been the inspiring stories of change from people who have turned their lives around.

All the best and good luck!
Michael

The Blood Sugar Diet: 50 Recipes

For the sake of simplicity, all calorie counts have been rounded up or down to the nearest 10 calories. All calorie counts are for one serving.

Breakfasts and Brunches

Yogurt with Passion Fruit and Almonds
Yogurt with Rhubarb Compote
Yogurt with Apple, Mango, and Hazelnuts
Almond Butter with Apple, Seeds, and Goji Berries
Portobello "Toast" with Wilted Spinach and Chickpeas
Portobello "Toast" with Goat Cheese and Pine Nuts
No-Carb Muesli
Spinach and Pea Omelet
Melon, Blueberry, and Spinach Smoothie
Grilled Apricots with Yogurt
Mango, Raspberry, and Lime Smoothie
Blueberry and Green Tea Smoothie
Spinach and Raspberry Green Drink
Vegetable Frittata
No-Carb Waffles
Baked Eggs with Minted Pea and Feta Salad
Poached Egg and Smoked Salmon Stack
Mexican Hash
Skinny Kedgeree

Soups, Salads, and Lunches

Crab and Mustard Lettuce Cups
Chicken and Walnut Lettuce Cups
Bacon and Avocado Lettuce Cups
Crayfish Salad
Beet Falafel
Pepper with Jeweled Feta
Zucchini and Feta Salad
Beet, Apple, and Cannellini Bean Soup
Chicken, Lima Bean, and Walnut Salad
Classic Spicy Hummus
Beet Hummus
Minted Pea Hummus
Spanish Chickpea and Spinach Soup
Chickpea and Hazelnut Salad
Shrimp Pho
Ricotta, Pear, and Walnut Salad
Skinny Spicy Bean Burgers
Chicken and Asparagus Salad
Grapefruit and Manchego Salad
Warm Halloumi Salad

Suppers

French Fish Stew
Luxury Fish Pie with Celeriac Topping
Zucchini Ribbons with Shrimp
Lamb and Pine Nut Meatballs with Moroccan Salad
Trout on Lime and Cilantro Crushed Peas
Pork with Apples and Shallots
Spicy Chicken and Lentils
Smoked Mackerel and Orange Salad

Eggplant with Lamb and Pomegranate
Steak with Crème Fraîche and Peppercorn Sauce
Harissa Chicken
Crab Cakes
Grilled Chicken on Cannellini Bean Mash
Stir-Fried Chicken with Lime and Coconut Milk
Spicy Turkey and Apricot Burgers with Salad
Foil-Steamed Fish
Skinny Chili
Braised Cod with Lettuce and Peas
Gingery Pork with Stir-Fried Vegetables

Quick and Easy

Five-Minute Breakfasts
Scrambled Eggs Three Ways
Cottage Cheese Three Ways
Avocado Three Ways

No-Fuss Lunches
Mediterranean Platter
Mexican Platter
No-Carb Ploughman's Lunch
Cheesy Baked Beans
Peanut Butter Dip
Sardine Dip

Simple Suppers
Five Ways to Jazz Up a Chicken Breast
Three Ways to Jazz Up a Salmon Steak
Three Ways to Jazz Up a Lamb Chop
Three Ways with Zucchini Ribbons
Three Ways with Cauliflower "Rice"
Three Quick Soups

Guilt-Free Baking

Zucchini and Pumpkin Seed Muffins
Cheesy Scones
Guilt-Free Brownies

Breakfasts

Yogurt with Passion Fruit and Almonds

170 CALORIES   SERVES 1

> 1 tablespoon sliced almonds
> 5 ounces plain yogurt
> 1 passion fruit

Toast the almonds in a dry skillet over low heat for a few minutes, until they turn golden. Remove them from the pan and allow them to cool.

Place the yogurt into a bowl and stir in the almonds. Cut the passion fruit in half, scoop out the seeds, and stir the seeds into the yogurt.

Yogurt with Rhubarb Compote

160 CALORIES   SERVES 1

>   1 pound rhubarb, trimmed and cut into small chunks
>   Zest and juice of 1 orange
>   Zest and juice of 1 lemon
>   1-inch piece fresh ginger, peeled and finely chopped
>   5 ounces plain yogurt

Preheat the oven to 350°F.

Put the rhubarb, zests, juices, and ginger in an ovenproof dish. Bake uncovered for 30 to 40 minutes. Allow to cool and then transfer to an airtight container. The rhubarb compote will keep in the fridge for 1 to 2 days.

To make the yogurt, swirl 2 tablespoons of the rhubarb compote through the yogurt.

Yogurt with Apple, Mango, and Hazelnuts

180 CALORIES   SERVES 1

>   ½ mango, peeled and cut into chunks
>   1 tablespoon hazelnuts, skins rubbed off
>   1 apple, cored and diced
>   5 ounces plain yogurt

Place the mango and hazelnuts in a food processor and pulse a few times to form a coarse paste. Place the paste in the bottom of a dish, add the chunks of apple, and top with the yogurt.

Almond Butter with Apple, Seeds, and Goji Berries

110 CALORIES   MAKES 4 SERVINGS

> 3½ ounces skin-on almonds
> 2 teaspoons mixed seeds and goji berries
> 1 apple, cored and sliced

To make the almond butter, preheat the oven to 375°F. Place the almonds on a baking sheet and bake for 10 minutes. Remove from the oven and allow to cool. Place in a food processor and process until smooth.

Serve 2 tablespoons of the almond butter in a dish and sprinkle with the seeds and goji berries. Add the apple wedges for dipping. Leftovers can be stored in the refrigerator for 2 to 3 days.

Portobello "Toast" with Wilted Spinach and Chickpeas

150 CALORIES   SERVES 1

> 2 portobello mushrooms
> Drizzle of olive oil
> Salt and black pepper
> 2 handfuls spinach
> Pinch of nutmeg
> 2 tablespoons canned chickpeas, drained and rinsed
> Pinch of paprika

Preheat the broiler. Place the mushrooms on a baking sheet, drizzle with the oil, and season with a pinch of salt and plenty of pepper. Broil for 3 minutes. Meanwhile, place the spinach in a small pan with a splash of water, place over medium heat, and cook until wilted. Drain and sprinkle with the nutmeg. Place the chickpeas in a bowl, sprinkle with the paprika, and coarsely mash with a fork. Divide the spinach and chickpeas between the two mushrooms.

Portobello "Toast" with Goat Cheese and Pine Nuts

150 CALORIES   SERVES 1

>   2 portobello mushrooms
>   Drizzle of olive oil
>   Salt and black pepper
>   1½ ounces goat cheese
>   1 tablespoon pine nuts
>   1 handful snipped chives

Preheat the broiler. Place the mushrooms on a baking sheet, drizzle with the oil, and season with a pinch of salt and plenty of pepper. Broil for 3 minutes.

Remove the mushrooms from the broiler, top with the cheese, and sprinkle with the pine nuts. Return to the broiler for 2 minutes more. Remove from the broiler and sprinkle on the chives.

No-Carb Muesli

180 CALORIES   SERVES 1

>   1 tablespoon raisins
>   ¼ cup apple juice
>   2 tablespoons ground flaxseeds
>   2 tablespoons plain yogurt
>   Pinch of cinnamon
>   1 tablespoon walnut pieces

Place the raisins in a bowl and pour on the apple juice. Let chill in the refrigerator for at least 1 hour or overnight.

When ready to eat, mix the raisins with the ground flaxseeds and the yogurt and sprinkle with the cinnamon and walnuts.

Spinach and Pea Omelet

180 CALORIES   SERVES 1

    2 ounces frozen peas
    2 handfuls baby spinach
    2 eggs
    Salt and black pepper
    1 tablespoon snipped chives
    Drizzle of olive oil

Bring a pan of water to a boil and cook the peas for 4 minutes. Add the spinach, cook 1 minute more, and then drain well. Beat the eggs, season with salt and pepper, add the peas, spinach, and chives, and mix well. Heat the oil in a pan, add the egg mixture, and cook through.

Melon, Blueberry, and Spinach Smoothie

130 CALORIES   SERVES 1

    ¼ Galia melon, peeled, seeded, and chopped
    2 ounces blueberries
    7 ounces unsweetened almond milk
    2 handfuls baby spinach
    Sprinkle of sunflower seeds

Put the melon, berries, and almond milk into a blender and whizz until smooth. Pour into a container.

Chill in the refrigerator for at least 1 hour or overnight.

Grilled Apricots with Yogurt

140 CALORIES   SERVES 2

>   1 teaspoon olive oil
>   1 tablespoon fresh lime juice
>   1 teaspoon cinnamon
>   6 apricots, peeled and cut into half-inch slices
>   4 tablespoons Greek yogurt
>   2 ounces raspberries
>   1 tablespoon hazelnuts, coarsely chopped
>   1 handful mint, torn

In a small bowl, combine the oil, lime juice, and cinnamon and whisk to blend.

Preheat the broiler. Lightly brush the apricots with the oil mixture. Broil, turning once and basting once or twice with the remaining marinade, until tender and golden, 3 to 5 minutes on each side.

Serve with the yogurt, scattered with the raspberries, hazelnuts, and mint.

Mango, Raspberry, and Lime Smoothie

150 CALORIES   SERVES 1

>   ½ mango, peeled, seeded, and chopped
>   2 ounces raspberries
>   2 handfuls baby spinach
>   1 teaspoon chia seeds
>   Juice of 1 lime
>   7 ounces coconut water

Place all the ingredients in a blender and whizz together.

Blueberry and Green Tea Smoothie

100 CALORIES   SERVES 1

> 7 ounces water
> 1 teabag green tea
> 2 ounces blueberries
> 2 tablespoons Greek yogurt
> 1 tablespoon almonds
> 1 tablespoon flaxseeds

Bring the water to a boil, add the teabag, and allow it to steep for 4 minutes. Remove the teabag and chill the tea in the fridge, preferably overnight. Place in a blender with the other ingredients and whizz together.

Spinach and Raspberry Green Drink

70 CALORIES   SERVES 1

> 2 large handfuls baby spinach
> 7 ounces coconut water
> 1 cup raspberries
> Juice of 1 lime

Combine the spinach and coconut water in a blender and blend. Add the berries and lime juice and blend again. Can be frozen, or stored in the fridge for 1 day.

Brunches

Vegetable Frittata

320 CALORIES   SERVES 2

 2 red bell peppers
 Olive oil
 3 scallions, chopped
 2 garlic cloves, crushed
 7 ounces canned chickpeas, drained and rinsed
 1 teaspoon smoked paprika
 3½ ounces baby spinach
 4 eggs, beaten
 Salt and black pepper

Stem the bell peppers and remove the seeds and ribs. Cut the peppers into halves or quarters. Brush lightly with oil, then place skin side up on a baking sheet and broil until the skin blackens and blisters. Place the hot peppers in a paper bag and seal tightly; let cool. When cooled, peel the charred skin from the peppers and coarsely chop the flesh.

Heat a drizzle of oil in a large ovenproof skillet over medium heat and sauté the scallions and garlic until soft. Add the bell peppers to the pan with the chickpeas and paprika. Sauté for about 5 minutes.

Add the spinach and keep stirring until it wilts. Add the eggs, season with salt and black pepper, and stir gently to incorporate the eggs into the whole mixture. Cook until set, about 2 minutes.

Slide the pan under a preheated broiler until the top of the frittata is light golden and puffed, about 1 minute.

177

No-Carb Waffles

290 CALORIES   MAKES 1 SERVING

> 2 egg whites plus 1 whole egg
> 2 tablespoons coconut flour
> 2 tablespoons milk
> ½ teaspoon baking powder
> Strawberries

Whip the egg whites to stiff peaks. Stir in the whole egg, coconut flour, milk, and baking powder. Heat a waffle iron to the highest temperature and grease it or spray it with nonstick spray. Pour in half the batter and cook until browned, 3 to 4 minutes. (If you don't have a waffle iron, use a hot skillet; spray the pan with oil and then use a ladle to pour half the mixture to make a thick pancake.) Repeat to make the second waffle. Serve with the strawberries.

Baked Eggs with Minted Pea and Feta Salad

330 CALORIES   SERVES 4

> 3 eggs
> 4½ fluid ounces half-fat crème fraîche
> 1 tablespoon grated Parmesan cheese
> 1 handful fresh basil, torn
> Salt and black pepper
> 10 ounces peas
> 3 tablespoons chopped fresh mint
> 1 avocado, peeled, seeded, and diced
> Juice of 1 lemon
> 1 tablespoon olive oil
> 2 ounces baby spinach
> 3½ ounces feta, crumbled

Preheat the oven to 350°F. Butter 4 cups of a muffin pan.

Whisk the eggs, crème fraîche, Parmesan, and basil in a bowl until well combined. Season to taste with salt and pepper. Divide the egg mixture among the muffin cups and bake in the oven for 10 to 12 minutes, until the eggs are just set.

Meanwhile, mix the peas, mint, avocado, lemon juice, and oil in a bowl.

To serve, divide the spinach onto 4 plates and spoon some pea and mint salad on top. Sprinkle with the feta and serve with the baked eggs.

Poached Egg and Smoked Salmon Stack

320 CALORIES   SERVES 2

> 4 portobello mushrooms
> Olive oil
> Salt and black pepper
> 2 ounces sliced smoked salmon
> 1 tablespoon half-fat crème fraîche
> 1 teaspoon grainy mustard
> Squeeze of lemon juice
> 2 handfuls watercress, chopped
> 2 eggs, poached
> 1 tablespoon pine nuts, toasted

Preheat the broiler. Place the mushrooms on a baking sheet, drizzle with the oil, and season with a pinch of salt and plenty of pepper. Broil for 3 minutes. Put a slice of smoked salmon on each mushroom. Mix the crème fraîche, mustard, and lemon juice and spread over the salmon. Top with a handful of watercress, a poached egg, and a scattering of pine nuts.

Mexican Hash

340 CALORIES   SERVES 2

> 1 red chile, slit lengthways and seeded
> 1 tablespoon canola oil
> 7 ounces baby mushrooms, halved
> 1 garlic clove, chopped
> 1 teaspoon Cajun seasoning
> 7 ounces canned black beans, drained and rinsed
> Salt and black pepper
> 2 eggs
> 1 ripe avocado, chopped
> Lime wedges

Slice half the chile into strips and set aside; finely chop the other half.

Heat half the oil in a pan over medium heat and sauté the mushrooms for about 5 minutes, until golden. Add the chopped chile, garlic, Cajun seasoning, and black beans and heat through for about 5 minutes; season to taste with salt and pepper. Keep warm.

In the same pan, heat the remaining oil and fry the eggs until cooked to your liking. Divide the mushroom mixture between two bowls and top each one with a fried egg, half the avocado, and half the chile strips. Serve with lime wedges.

Skinny Kedgeree

360 CALORIES   SERVES 2

> 1 large cauliflower
> 1 tablespoon olive oil
> 2 eggs
> 1 small red onion, chopped
> 1 red chile, seeded and chopped
> 2 tablespoons medium-hot curry powder
> 1 teaspoon mustard seeds
> 1 teaspoon cayenne pepper
> 2 small smoked mackerel fillets, flaked
> Salt and black pepper
> 4 scallions, sliced
> 1 handful flat-leaf parsley, chopped

To make cauliflower "rice," preheat the oven to 400°F. Cut the cauliflower into florets, place in a food processor, and process for 30 seconds. Transfer into a bowl, drizzle with half the oil, and toss gently. Spread the cauliflower in a thin layer on a baking sheet and bake for 10 minutes.

In a small pan, boil the eggs for 7 minutes.

Meanwhile, heat the remaining oil in a nonstick skillet over medium heat and sauté the onion and chile for 5 minutes, until soft. Add the curry powder, mustard seeds, and cayenne and sauté for 1 to 2 minutes more.

Stir the cauliflower rice into the onion mixture and then add the mackerel. Season well with salt and black pepper and heat through gently.

Peel and quarter the boiled eggs. Stir the scallions and parsley into the rice mixture, divide between two bowls, and top with the egg quarters.

Soups, Salads, and Lunches

Crab and Mustard Lettuce Cups

210 CALORIES   SERVES 1

>1 tablespoon crème fraîche
>1 teaspoon Dijon mustard
>Squeeze of lemon juice
>3½ ounces white crabmeat
>1 small handful chopped dill
>1 teaspoon capers
>Lettuce leaves

Blend the crème fraîche, mustard, and lemon juice. Add the crabmeat, dill, and capers, and mix well. Serve on the lettuce leaves.

Chicken and Walnut Lettuce Cups

300 CALORIES   SERVES 1

>1 tablespoon crème fraîche
>1 teaspoon Dijon mustard
>Squeeze of lemon juice
>3½ ounces cooked chicken, chopped
>1 small red apple, cored and sliced
>1 tablespoon chopped walnuts
>1 celery stalk, chopped
>Lettuce leaves

Blend the crème fraîche, mustard, and lemon juice. Add the chicken pieces, apple, walnuts, and celery and mix well. Serve on lettuce leaves.

Bacon and Avocado Lettuce Cups

290 CALORIES   SERVES 1

> 2 strips lean bacon, cooked and cut into thin strips
> 1 radish, diced
> ½ avocado, peeled, seeded, and chopped
> Lettuce leaves

Combine the bacon, radish, and avocado. Serve on lettuce leaves.

Crayfish Salad

250 CALORIES   SERVES 1

> 1 small shallot
> 1 garlic clove
> ½ red chile
> 1 tablespoon olive oil
> 1 tablespoon fish sauce
> Juice of 1 lemon
> 1 tablespoon white wine vinegar
> 3½ ounces crayfish
> 4 radishes, halved
> ½ cucumber, diced
> 1 stalk celery, chopped
> 2 large handfuls arugula

Make the dressing: Finely chop the shallot, garlic, and chile. Place in a jar with the oil, fish sauce, lemon juice, and vinegar. Cover and shake well. (You will have extra dressing.)

Arrange the crayfish in a bowl with the radishes, cucumber, celery, and arugula and dress with 1 tablespoon of the dressing.

Beet Falafel

290 CALORIES   SERVES 2

½ tablespoon olive oil
1 red onion, chopped
1 teaspoon cumin seeds
Pinch of cayenne pepper
4 mushrooms, finely chopped
14 ounces canned chickpeas, drained and rinsed
9 ounces beets, peeled and coarsely grated
1 egg
1 tablespoon tahini
Squeeze of lemon juice
Salt and black pepper
Vegetable oil
2 tablespoons Greek yogurt
1 bag arugula

Preheat the oven to 400°F.

Heat the oil in a skillet and sauté the onions for 5 minutes, until softened. Add the cumin, cayenne, and mushrooms and cook for another 2 minutes. Transfer the mixture to a food processor and add the chickpeas, two-thirds of the grated beets, egg, tahini, and lemon juice. Process to a coarse paste. Transfer to a bowl and stir in the remaining grated beets. Season with a pinch of salt and plenty of black pepper.

With wet hands, shape into eight balls and space on a baking sheet lined with parchment. Brush the falafels with a little oil and bake for 25 minutes.

Serve the falafels with a dollop of Greek yogurt and a handful of arugula.

Pepper with Jeweled Feta

220 CALORIES   SERVES 1

1 red bell pepper

Olive oil

1 ounce feta, diced

1 tablespoon chopped mint

1 tablespoon chopped
  cilantro

1 scallion, finely chopped

1 tablespoon chopped
  pistachios

4 cherry tomatoes, halved

2-inch piece cucumber,
  diced

Seeds from 1 pomegranate

Juice of ½ lemon

Preheat the broiler. Halve the bell pepper and remove the seeds. Brush the skin with the oil and place skin side up on a baking tray. Broil the pepper for 5 minutes.

Combine all the other ingredients in a bowl.

Remove the bell pepper halves from the broiler and stuff with the feta mixture.

Zucchini and Feta Salad

270 CALORIES   SERVES 1

1 zucchini

2 large handfuls arugula

2 ounces raspberries

1 tablespoon olive oil

1 tablespoon balsamic vinegar

1½ ounces feta, diced

1 tablespoon pumpkin seeds

1 handful mint, torn

Peel a zucchini into long ribbons using a spiralizer or potato peeler. Mix with the arugula and raspberries. Drizzle with the oil and vinegar and top with the feta, pumpkin seeds, and mint.

Beet, Apple, and Cannellini Bean Soup

200 CALORIES   SERVES 3

    1 tablespoon olive oil
    1 teaspoon cumin seeds
    2 medium onions, coarsely chopped
    1 pound beets, grated
    2 cooking apples, peeled, cored, and quartered
    1 quart chicken or vegetable stock
    2 star anise
    Salt and black pepper
    14 ounces cannellini beans, drained and rinsed
    Greek yogurt
    Handful of chives, chopped

Heat the oil in a large saucepan over medium heat, then add the cumin seeds and onions, cover, and cook gently for 10 minutes. Add the beets and the apples, stir well, cover, and cook for another 10 minutes. Pour in the stock, turn up the heat, add the star anise, and season with a pinch of salt and plenty of pepper. Bring to a boil, then reduce the heat and simmer for 5 minutes. Remove from the heat and remove the star anise. Transfer the soup to a blender and puree. Return the soup to the pan, add the beans, and simmer for 20 minutes. Serve with a swirl of Greek yogurt and some chives. Leftovers can be stored in the refrigerator for 2 to 3 days or frozen for a month.

Chicken, Lima Bean, and Walnut Salad

270 CALORIES   SERVES 2

    7 ounces diced chicken breast
    Leaves from 2 sprigs rosemary, finely chopped
    1 garlic clove, finely chopped
    Olive oil

2 ounces green beans, trimmed
3½ ounces canned lima beans, drained and rinsed
1 red onion, very thinly sliced
1 tablespoon chopped walnut pieces
1 tablespoon grainy mustard
1 tablespoon white wine vinegar

Place the chicken, rosemary, and garlic in a large bowl. Drizzle with a little oil and toss together.

Place a large nonstick skillet over medium-high heat and add the chicken. Cook, stirring, for about 10 minutes until the chicken is browned on all sides and cooked through.

Meanwhile, bring a large pan of water to a boil and add the green beans. Boil for 2 minutes, then add the lima beans and cook for another 2 minutes, until the green beans are tender and the lima beans are heated through. Drain well.

In a large serving bowl, mix the warm chicken, beans, onion, and walnuts. Whisk together 1 tablespoon of oil with mustard and vinegar to make a dressing; pour over and toss gently to combine.

Classic Spicy Hummus

250 CALORIES   SERVES 3

14 ounces canned chickpeas, drained and rinsed
Juice of ½ lemon
1 garlic clove
1 teaspoon paprika
2 tablespoons olive oil
2 tablespoons tahini

Combine all the ingredients in a food processor and process until smooth. If it is too thick, add a little water. Leftovers will keep in the refrigerator for 2 to 3 days.

Beet Hummus

200 CALORIES   SERVES 3

> 9 ounces beets
> 28 ounces canned chickpeas, drained and rinsed
> Juice of 1 lemon
> 1 teaspoon ground cumin
> Salt and black pepper
> 2 tablespoons Greek yogurt

Cook the beets in a large pan of boiling water, covered, for 30 to 40 minutes, until tender. When they're done, a skewer or knife should go all the way in easily. Drain, then set aside to cool.

When cool enough to handle, peel and coarsely chop the flesh. Place the beets in a food processor along with the chickpeas, lemon juice, cumin, a pinch of salt, and some pepper. Process until smooth. Transfer to a bowl and swirl in the yogurt. Leftovers will keep in the refrigerator for 2 to 3 days.

Minted Pea Hummus

170 CALORIES   SERVES 3

> 8½ ounces cooked peas
> 1 garlic clove, crushed
> 1 tablespoon tahini
> Squeeze of lemon juice
> 1 tablespoon canned chickpeas
> 2 tablespoons olive oil
> 1 handful mint

Place all the ingredients in a food processor and process to form a thick paste. Add 1 to 2 tablespoons water, then process again. Leftovers will keep in the refrigerator for 2 to 3 days.

Spanish Chickpea and Spinach Soup

210 CALORIES   SERVES 2

2 ounces Spanish chorizo, diced
1 tablespoon olive oil
1 large leek, rinsed well and thinly sliced
2 garlic cloves, finely chopped
1 red bell pepper, diced
Pinch of red pepper flakes
1 teaspoon paprika
1 tablespoon tomato puree
1 quart chicken stock
7 ounces canned chickpeas, drained and rinsed
5 ounces baby spinach

Place a small nonstick pan over medium heat and add the chorizo; allow to cook, stirring occasionally, for about 5 minutes, until most of the fat melts out. Set aside to drain on paper towels. Discard the fat.

Heat the oil in a large pan over medium heat. Add the leek and cook, stirring frequently, for about 5 minutes, until just soft. Add the garlic, bell pepper, red pepper flakes, and paprika and cook for 1 minute. Add the tomato puree and cook, stirring frequently, for 2 minutes more. Add the stock and chickpeas and bring to a boil. Reduce the heat to a simmer, partially cover, and cook for 20 minutes.

Finally, add the spinach and chorizo and heat through for 2 minutes, until the spinach is wilted.

Chickpea and Hazelnut Salad

270 CALORIES   SERVES 2

    3½ ounces peeled and diced butternut squash
    1 tablespoon olive oil
    ½ teaspoon allspice
    7 ounces canned chickpeas, drained and rinsed
    1 tablespoon hazelnuts
    3 ounces green beans
    2 handfuls watercress
    8 cherry tomatoes, halved
    2 scallions, chopped
    ½ cucumber, chopped
    1 tablespoon balsamic vinegar

Preheat the oven to 375°F. Place the butternut squash in a pan, cover with boiling water, and simmer for 5 minutes, drain well, and then spread out on a baking sheet. Drizzle with half the oil, sprinkle with allspice, and bake for 15 minutes, until golden.

Transfer the butternut squash to a bowl and add the chickpeas, hazelnuts, green beans, watercress, tomatoes, scallions, and cucumber. Toss and dress with the remaining oil and the vinegar.

Shrimp Pho

170 CALORIES   MAKES 2 PORTIONS

    1 quart vegetable stock
    1 handful bean sprouts
    2 ounces snow peas
    2 ounces sugar snap peas
    2 ounces baby corn
    1-inch piece ginger, peeled and grated
    1 tablespoon fish sauce
    Juice of ½ lime

12 large shrimp, shelled and deveined
1 handful each fresh basil, mint, and cilantro
½ red chile, finely sliced

Pour the stock into a large saucepan and bring to a boil. Add the bean sprouts, snow peas, sugar snap peas, baby corn, and ginger and cook for 3 to 4 minutes. Add the fish sauce and lime juice. Add the shrimp and cook until pink, 2 to 3 minutes. Serve topped with the herbs and chile.

Ricotta, Pear, and Walnut Salad

290 CALORIES   SERVES 1

2 ounces fresh ricotta
2 scallions, finely chopped
2 ounces green beans
1 tablespoon olive oil
1 tablespoon lemon juice
½ garlic clove, crushed
1 handful flat-leaf parsley, chopped
Pinch of nutmeg
Salt and black pepper
2 large handfuls watercress
1 small pear
1 tablespoon chopped walnuts

Crumble the ricotta into a bowl, add the scallions, and toss gently. Place the green beans into a small pan of boiling water and cook for 3 to 4 minutes; drain well, rinse under cold running water, and set aside. Make the salad dressing by whisking the oil, lemon juice, garlic, parsley, and nutmeg in a bowl. Season with salt and pepper. Arrange the watercress, green beans, and pear in a dish, add the ricotta and scallion mixture, drizzle with the dressing, and top with walnuts.

Skinny Spicy Bean Burgers

280 CALORIES   SERVES 2

 4 mushrooms
 1 handful cilantro
 14 ounces canned cannellini beans, drained and rinsed
 14 ounces canned kidney beans, drained and rinsed
 1 egg
 ½ onion, finely chopped
 1 chile, finely sliced
 1 teaspoon coriander
 1 teaspoon cumin
 1 teaspoon paprika
 1 teaspoon chili powder or a few drops of Tabasco sauce
 Flour
 Olive oil
 Bag of salad greens
 1 tomato, sliced

Place the mushrooms and cilantro in a food processor and process until the mixture resembles bread crumbs. Add the beans and egg and blend together to form a chunky mixture.

Stir in the rest of the ingredients. Dust your hands with flour and shape the mixture into 4 burger patties.

Heat a drizzle of oil in a large pan and fry the burgers over medium heat until brown and hot all the way through. Serve with handfuls of salad greens and thick slices of the tomato.

Chicken and Asparagus Salad

270 CALORIES   SERVES 2

2 skinless, boneless chicken breasts
1 bundle asparagus (about 7 ounces), tough ends snapped off
    and discarded
1 red bell pepper, seeds and ribs removed, and thinly sliced
Olive oil
Salt and black pepper
2 tablespoons yogurt
1 tablespoon sour cream
1 tablespoon white wine vinegar
1 tablespoon chopped dill
½ garlic clove, crushed
4½ ounces mixed salad greens
2 tablespoons pine nuts, toasted

Preheat the oven to 425°F. Arrange the chicken, asparagus, and bell pepper in a large, shallow roasting pan and drizzle with oil; toss to coat. Season with salt and black pepper and roast in the oven for 20 minutes, stirring halfway through, until the chicken is cooked through and the vegetables are tender and starting to caramelize.

In a small bowl, whisk the yogurt, sour cream, vinegar, dill, and garlic to make a dressing. Season to taste.

Divide the salad greens between two plates, scatter with pine nuts, and arrange the chicken and vegetables on top. Serve with the dressing.

Grapefruit and Manchego Salad

280 CALORIES   SERVES 2

> 1 large pink grapefruit
> 3 ounces Manchego cheese (or cheddar), diced
> 1 avocado, peeled and diced
> ½ bulb fennel, thinly sliced
> Juice of 1 lime
> 1 tablespoon olive oil
> 1 tablespoon balsamic vinegar
> Large handful cilantro, chopped

Peel the grapefruit and separate the segments with a knife, catching the juice in a bowl. Combine the cheese, avocado, fennel, grapefruit sections, and juice in a bowl and toss. To make the dressing, whisk the lime juice, oil, and vinegar. Pour the dressing over the salad and sprinkle with cilantro.

Warm Halloumi Salad

280 CALORIES   SERVES 2

> ½ teaspoon chili powder
> 1 large handful mint, chopped
> Zest and juice of ½ lemon
> 1 tablespoon olive oil
> 1 zucchini, cut into ½-inch rounds
> 5 ounces halloumi cheese, cubed
> 4 handfuls arugula
> 1 red bell pepper, diced
> 1 tablespoon sliced black olives

Mix the chili powder, half the mint, the lemon zest and lemon juice, oil, zucchini, and halloumi. Let marinate for 30 minutes. Soak 8 wooden skewers in water for 20 minutes.

Thread the zucchini and halloumi onto the skewers, put the remaining marinade to one side. Grill or broil for 7 to 8 minutes, turning halfway through, and basting with a bit of the remaining marinade.

Place the arugula in a bowl with the bell pepper, olives, remaining mint and dress with the last of the marinade.

Suppers X 18
(Approximately 350 to 500 Calories)

French Fish Stew

390 CALORIES   SERVES 2

> Olive oil
> 1 shallot, finely chopped
> 1 fennel bulb, finely chopped
> 1 garlic clove, finely chopped
> Vermouth or dry white wine
> 10½ ounces chicken stock
> 7 ounces canned tomatoes
> 9 ounces mixed fresh seafood (shrimp, crab, white fish,
>   crayfish, etc.)
> 2 to 3 handfuls baby spinach
> Salt and black pepper

Heat a drizzle of oil in a large pan. Add the shallot, fennel, and garlic and cook for 5 minutes, until softened. Add a splash of vermouth and let bubble for a minute. Pour in the stock and tomatoes and bring to a boil. Simmer for 15 minutes. Stir in the seafood and spinach, and cook until the seafood is cooked through. Season to taste.

Luxury Fish Pie with Celeriac Topping

470 CALORIES   SERVES 4

    2 small celeriac roots, peeled and diced
    8½ ounces plus 1 tablespoon milk
    1 tablespoon butter
    Salt and black pepper
    Olive oil
    1 large onion, finely diced
    2 leeks, finely sliced
    2 tablespoons chopped flat-leaf parsley
    1 tablespoon chopped fresh dill
    3½ ounces mushrooms, chopped
    14 ounces sustainable white fish fillets (haddock or cod),
       cut into chunks
    5 ounces peeled shrimp
    1 bay leaf

Preheat the oven to 350°F.

Boil the celeriac for about 10 minutes, until tender. Drain and transfer to a food processor. Add 1 tablespoon milk, the butter, some salt and pepper and puree. Set aside.

Heat a drizzle of oil in a large pan and cook the onion, leeks, parsley, and dill for a few minutes, until softened. Transfer to a plate. In the same pan, cook the mushrooms for a few minutes until lightly golden. Add to the reserved onion and leeks.

Place the fish and shrimp into a large pan, add the remaining milk and bay leaf, and bring to a boil. Reduce the heat to a simmer and poach for about 4 minutes. Remove the fish and shrimp from the pan and put aside; reserve the milk, removing any bones or skin and the bay leaf.

Arrange the fish and shrimp in an ovenproof serving dish. Layer the mushrooms and the onion and leek mixture on top. Drizzle with 3 to 4 tablespoons of the reserved cooking milk.

Cover with the mashed celeriac. Bake for 15 minutes.

Zucchini Ribbons with Shrimp

390 CALORIES   SERVES 2

> 1 large or 2 small leeks, thickly sliced
> 1 zucchini, spiralized or cut into ribbons with a peeler
> 1-inch piece of fresh ginger, peeled and grated
> ½ red chile, chopped
> 1 garlic clove, crushed
> Juice of 1 lemon
> 1 tablespoon olive oil
> 7 ounces shrimp
> 7 ounces canned cannellini beans, drained and rinsed
> Salt and black pepper
> 2 handfuls cilantro, chopped

Steam the leeks for 4 to 5 minutes, until tender, adding the zucchini for the final 2 minutes. Set aside.

Using a food processor or a mortar and pestle, make a paste with the ginger, chile, garlic, and lemon juice. Heat the oil in a pan over medium heat, add the paste, and sauté for a couple of minutes.

Add the shrimp and beans and cook for 10 minutes, until the shrimp are pink and cooked through. Add the leeks and zucchini to the pan and toss. Season with salt and pepper and then top with the cilantro before serving.

Lamb and Pine Nut Meatballs with Moroccan Salad

480 CALORIES   SERVES 2

>   7 ounces ground lamb
>   1 small onion, finely grated
>   2 garlic cloves, crushed
>   2 ounces pine nuts, lightly toasted and coarsely chopped
>   ½ teaspoon paprika
>   ¼ teaspoon ground allspice
>   ½ teaspoon ground cumin
>   1 egg white, lightly whisked
>   1 small bunch flat-leaf parsley, finely chopped
>   1 small bunch mint, finely chopped
>   Salt and black pepper
>   1 tablespoon vegetable oil
>   3½ ounces baby spinach
>   1 tablespoon sliced almonds
>   ½ cucumber, peeled, seeded, and cut into small chunks
>   2 tablespoons chickpeas, drained and rinsed
>   2 scallions, chopped
>   1 teaspoon olive oil
>   1 tablespoon balsamic vinegar
>   Juice of half a lemon

In a large bowl, mix the lamb, onion, garlic, pine nuts, paprika, allspice, and cumin. Add the egg white and mix again. Stir in the parsley and mint and season to taste with salt and pepper. Shape the mixture into six evenly sized balls.

Heat the vegetable oil in a skillet and fry the meatballs over medium heat, turning occasionally, for 10 minutes, until browned on all sides and completely cooked through.

Place the spinach in a bowl. Add the almonds, cucumber, chickpeas, and scallions; drizzle with the olive oil and vinegar, and toss. Serve with the meatballs.

Trout on Lime and Cilantro Crushed Peas

480 CALORIES   SERVES 2

> 9 ounces trout fillets
> Olive oil
> 2 limes, 1 peeled and sliced, the other juiced
> ½ teaspoon ground cumin
> Salt and black pepper
> 7 ounces frozen peas
> 1 tablespoon Greek yogurt
> Large handful cilantro, finely chopped

Preheat the oven to 350°F.

Lay the trout fillets in an ovenproof dish and drizzle with oil. Top the fish with the lime slices, sprinkle with the cumin, season with salt and pepper, and place in the oven to roast for 8 minutes, or until cooked through.

Meanwhile, cook the peas in boiling water for 3 minutes until tender. Drain and place in a bowl. Add the yogurt and lime juice and use a potato masher to crush the peas into a coarse mash. Stir in most of the cilantro and season with salt and pepper.

Serve the trout on top of the mashed peas and sprinkle with the remaining cilantro.

Pork with Apples and Shallots

450 CALORIES   SERVES 8

> 1 (8-pound) rolled boneless pork roast
> 8 garlic cloves, crushed
> 1 bunch fresh sage, finely chopped
> Salt and black pepper
> 5 tablespoons olive oil
> 2 large leeks, diagonally sliced
> 16 shallots
> 6 small apples, cored and cut into quarters
> 1 tablespoon butter
> 1 cup apple cider

Preheat the oven to 475°F. Unroll the pork and score the flesh with a sharp knife.

Make a paste with the garlic, sage, a pinch of salt and pepper, and 3 tablespoons of the oil and spread it over the meat. Roll the pork back up and tie it with kitchen twine.

Place the leeks in the bottom of a roasting dish, toss with the remaining 2 tablespoons oil, then lay the pork on top and roast for about 25 minutes.

Meanwhile, in a skillet, brown the shallots and apple wedges in the butter.

Turn the oven down to 350°F. Place the shallots and apple wedges around the pork and roast for another 45 minutes to 1 hour, until a meat thermometer inserted into the thickest part of the meat reads 165° to 170°F.

Remove the pork, apples, and shallots from the oven and keep warm.

Strain the pan juices into a small saucepan, add the cider, and bring to a boil. Reduce to a simmer and cook until slightly thickened. Slice the pork and serve with apples, shallots, and gravy.

Spicy Chicken and Lentils

470 CALORIES   SERVES 1

½ bulb fennel, thinly sliced
½ red onion, cut into thin wedges
1 garlic clove, crushed
1 handful fresh thyme
Olive oil
Pinch of red pepper flakes
1 skinless, boneless chicken breast
7 ounces vegetable stock
7 ounces canned green lentils
Salt and black pepper
2 ounces snow peas

Preheat the oven to 400°F. Place the fennel, onion, garlic, and thyme in a roasting pan, drizzle with a little oil, and sprinkle with red pepper flakes. Place the chicken breast on top. Roast for 20 minutes, then remove from the oven and turn down the temperature to 300°F.

Add the stock and lentils to the roasting pan and stir in around the chicken. Season with salt and black pepper, then return to the oven for another 20 minutes.

Meanwhile, steam or boil the snow peas for 3 to 4 minutes. Serve the chicken with the snow peas.

Smoked Mackerel and Orange Salad

460 CALORIES   SERVES 2

> 7 ounces small beets
> 2 tablespoons red wine vinegar
> Zest and juice of ½ orange
> 1 tablespoon olive oil
> Salt and black pepper
> 2 oranges
> 1 head endive
> 2 scallions, sliced diagonally
> 2 small smoked mackerel fillets
> 1 ounce walnut halves

Preheat the oven to 400°F. Put the beets in a roasting pan with ¾ inch of water in the bottom. Cover with foil and roast for 30 minutes.

Meanwhile, put the vinegar, orange zest and juice, and oil into a jar, season with salt and pepper, cover, and shake until well combined.

Remove the beets from the oven (they should be tender when pierced with a knife). When they are cool enough to handle, peel off the skins and slice the beets into rounds. Toss them in a little of the dressing.

Peel the oranges, following the contour of the fruit, then cut each one into thin slices. Trim the endive and separate the leaves, discarding the outer ones.

Arrange the endive leaves in a salad bowl and then add the beets, orange slices, and scallions. Flake the fish on top, add the walnuts, and drizzle with the remaining dressing.

Eggplant with Lamb and Pomegranate

490 CALORIES   SERVES 2

> 2 eggplants, halved lengthwise
> 1 tablespoon olive oil
> Salt and black pepper
> 1 onion, finely chopped
> ½ teaspoon ground cumin
> ½ teaspoon paprika
> ½ teaspoon cinnamon
> 7 ounces lean ground lamb
> 1 tablespoon pine nuts
> 1 tablespoon tomato puree
> 2 tablespoons pomegranate seeds
> 1 handful flat-leaf parsley, chopped

Preheat the oven to 425°F. Place the eggplant in a roasting dish skin side down. Lightly brush with some of the oil, season with a pinch of salt and plenty of pepper, and bake in the oven for 20 minutes.

Meanwhile, heat the remaining oil in a pan, add the onion, cumin, paprika, and cinnamon and cook over medium heat for 8 minutes. Add the lamb, pine nuts, and tomato puree and cook for 8 minutes more. Just before the end of the cooking time, stir in the pomegranate seeds.

Remove the eggplant from the oven and divide the lamb mixture evenly between each half. Return to the oven and bake 10 minutes more. Serve topped with parsley.

Steak with Crème Fraîche and Peppercorn Sauce

510 CALORIES   SERVES 2

> 7 ounces beef stock
> 3½ ounces red wine
> Salt
> 2 sirloin steaks (8 ounces each)
> Pinch of steak seasoning
> 1 teaspoon butter
> 1 teaspoon olive oil
> 2 tablespoons crème fraîche
> 2 teaspoons mixed peppercorns, coarsely crushed
> Two large handfuls mixed greens

Pour the stock and wine into a small saucepan and boil rapidly for about 10 minutes to reduce it, then season with a pinch of salt.

Season the steaks with a pinch of steak seasoning and allow to reach room temperature. Place a skillet over high heat and add the butter and oil. Add the steaks to the hot pan and, keeping the heat high, cook 3 minutes on one side for medium or 2 minutes for rare. Turn them over and give them another 2 minutes on the other side for medium or 1 minute for rare.

Pour in the reduced stock, crème fraîche, and peppercorns. Stir well and cook for 1 minute more. Serve with mixed greens.

Harissa Chicken

420 CALORIES   SERVES 2

2 skinless, boneless chicken breasts
4 teaspoons harissa
1 tablespoon olive oil
Salt and black pepper
1 tablespoon pine nuts
4 large handfuls baby spinach
2 scallions, chopped
¼ cucumber, chopped
2 tomatoes, chopped
7 ounces canned navy beans, drained and rinsed
1 tablespoon raisins
1 handful flat-leaf parsley, chopped
1 handful mint, chopped

Preheat the oven to 325°F. Smear each chicken breast with 2 teaspoons harissa and place in an ovenproof dish. Drizzle with the oil, season with salt and pepper, and bake for 20 to 25 minutes, until cooked through. Remove from the oven, allow to cool slightly, and then shred the meat.

Put the pine nuts in a dry skillet and place over medium heat for a few minutes to toast, until golden.

Place the spinach in a bowl and add the scallions, cucumber, tomatoes, beans, raisins, parsley, and mint. Place the chicken on top and sprinkle with the pine nuts.

Crab Cakes

440 CALORIES   SERVES 1

    3½ ounces crabmeat
    1 tablespoon canned sweet corn, drained and rinsed
    Pinch of paprika
    Splash of Worcestershire sauce
    1 teaspoon mayonnaise
    1 scallion, chopped
    1 handful flat-leaf parsley, chopped
    Juice of ½ lemon
    Black pepper
    Flour
    Olive oil
    A couple of florets of broccoli, steamed

In a bowl, combine the crabmeat, corn, paprika, Worcestershire sauce, mayonnaise, scallion, and parsley. Stir in the lemon juice and season with pepper. Place the bowl in the fridge for a few hours.

Sprinkle some flour, seasoned with pepper, on a clean surface and on your hands and shape the crab mixture into 2 patties. Heat a drizzle of oil in a nonstick skillet and fry the crab cakes for 3 minutes on each side. Serve with the broccoli.

Grilled Chicken on Cannellini Bean Mash

440 CALORIES   SERVES 2

    2 skinless, boneless chicken breasts
    1 tablespoon olive oil
    Salt and black pepper
    1 shallot, finely chopped
    1 to 2 garlic cloves, chopped

14 ounces canned cannellini beans, drained and rinsed
Large handful flat-leaf parsley, chopped
Steamed green beans or broccoli

Drizzle a little of the oil onto the chicken breasts and season well with a pinch of salt and plenty of pepper. Grill the chicken breasts for 10 minutes, turning regularly.

Meanwhile, heat the remaining oil in a saucepan and add the shallot. Cook gently for 5 minutes, then add the garlic and cook for another 2 minutes, until soft. Add the cannellini beans to the pan and mash coarsely, adding a little stock or water if needed. Stir in the parsley and add salt and pepper.

Serve with the green beans or broccoli.

Stir-Fried Chicken with Lime and Coconut Milk

340 CALORIES   SERVES 2

2 teaspoons canola oil
2 skinless chicken breasts, chopped into 1-inch pieces
1 green chile, seeded and finely chopped
5 ounces coconut milk
1 tablespoon fish sauce
4 scallions, chopped
1 large handful cilantro, chopped
Juice of 1 lime

Heat the oil in a wok over high heat, add the chicken, and stir-fry for 5 minutes, until golden. Add the chile and stir-fry for 1 minute. Add the coconut milk, fish sauce, scallions, and cilantro. Cook for another 3 minutes, then serve, drizzled with the lime juice. You could also serve with 2 tablespoons cooked brown rice (adds 70 calories).

Spicy Turkey and Apricot Burgers with Salad

460 CALORIES   SERVES 2

5 mushrooms
9 ounces ground turkey
½ onion, finely chopped
6 dried apricots, finely chopped
1 tablespoon finely chopped flat-leaf parsley
1 teaspoon baharat
1 small egg, beaten
1 tablespoon olive oil
Salt and black pepper
3 scallions, chopped
3½ ounces arugula
2 ounces blanched almonds
2 ounces pomegranate seeds
3½ ounces cherry tomatoes, diced
Squeeze of lemon juice

Place the mushrooms in a food processer and process until they resemble breadcrumbs.

Combine the mushrooms, turkey, onion, apricots, parsley, baharat, and egg in a bowl, season with a pinch of salt and plenty of pepper, and mix with your hands. Form into evenly sized small balls.

Heat the oil in a skillet over high heat and sear the meatballs for 5 minutes, until browned on all sides. Reduce the heat and cook for another 10 minutes, until cooked through. Remove the meatballs and keep warm.

In the same pan, cook the scallions for 3 minutes.

Place the arugula in a bowl and toss with the cooked scallions. Add the almonds, pomegranate, and tomatoes, squeeze some lemon juice over, and then serve with the meatballs.

Foil-Steamed Fish

370 CALORIES   SERVES 2

> 2 pieces skinless fish fillet (halibut, cod, haddock, etc.),
>   4½ ounces each
> 2 tomatoes, chopped
> 4 scallions, trimmed and cut on the diagonal
> 1 red chile, seeded and sliced
> 1 carrot, peeled and julienned
> Juice of 1 lime
> 1 tablespoon soy sauce
> 3½ ounces green beans, trimmed
> 1 handful cilantro, chopped

Preheat the oven to 425°F. Place each fish fillet on a sheet of foil and put on a large baking sheet.

In a bowl, mix the tomatoes, scallions, chile, and carrot, then pile half of the mixture on top of each fish fillet. Divide the lime juice and soy sauce over them, and then wrap each fish fillet in the foil to make a parcel. Bake in the oven for 15 minutes.

Meanwhile, add the green beans to a pan of boiling water and allow to simmer for 4 to 5 minutes. Serve the fish with the beans, topped with cilantro.

Skinny Chili

460 CALORIES   SERVES 8

 1 pound mushrooms
 2 tablespoons canola oil
 1 pound lean ground beef
 2 red onions, finely chopped
 2 stalks celery, chopped
 1½ to 3 teaspoons crushed red pepper flakes
 1½ teaspoons ground cumin
 1½ teaspoons dried oregano
 28 ounces canned chopped tomatoes
 17 ounces beef or vegetable stock
 14 ounces canned kidney beans, drained and rinsed
 14 ounces canned black-eyed peas, drained and rinsed
 1 cinnamon stick
 Salt and black pepper
 3 ounces plain chocolate, coarsely chopped
 1 handful cilantro, chopped
 Greek yogurt

Preheat the oven to 300°F. Place the mushrooms in a food processor and process until they resemble ground meat. Heat half the oil over medium-high heat in a large flameproof casserole. Add the beef and fry until browned all over. Remove from the pan with a slotted spoon and set aside.

Add the remaining oil to the pan and cook the onions and celery for 3 to 4 minutes, until softened. Stir in the mushrooms, red pepper flakes, cumin, and oregano. Cook for 3 minutes.

Return the beef to the pan, then stir in the tomatoes, stock, kidney beans, and black-eyed peas. Snap the cinnamon stick in half and add to the pan. Bring to a boil, then reduce the heat and cover tightly. Place in the oven and cook for 2 to 3 hours.

Remove from the oven and taste and adjust the seasoning. Stir in the chocolate pieces until they have just melted, then scatter with the chopped cilantro. Serve with the yogurt.

Braised Cod with Lettuce and Peas

440 CALORIES   SERVES 1

>3½ ounces frozen peas
>1 small head lettuce (Gem, butter, or romaine), shredded
>1 tablespoon olive oil
>5 ounces boneless cod or white fish fillets
>Salt and black pepper
>2 scallions, thickly sliced
>1 tablespoon crème fraîche
>Juice of ½ lemon

Place the peas in a pan of boiling water and cook for 5 minutes. Add the lettuce and cook for 2 minutes more. Drain well in a colander and then place the colander on top of the empty pan and put back on the heat for 1 minute; this allows the peas and lettuce to steam for a bit to remove any excess water.

Heat the oil in a large pan over medium heat. Season the cod well with salt and pepper and place it in the pan. Add the scallions and cook for 3 to 4 minutes on each side.

Add the lettuce, peas, crème fraîche, and lemon juice to the pan and cook for 2 minutes more, until heated through.

Gingery Pork with Stir-Fried Vegetables

270 CALORIES   SERVES 2

  1 tablespoon soy sauce
  2 tablespoons red wine vinegar
  2 garlic cloves, crushed
  1 tablespoon grated ginger
  2 lean pork fillets (approximately 4½ ounces each)
  1 teaspoon canola oil
  1 medium onion, sliced
  1 small carrot, finely sliced
  1 zucchini, sliced
  2 teaspoons cornstarch
  5 ounces snow peas, halved
  3½ ounces bean sprouts

Combine the soy sauce, vinegar, garlic, and ginger in a bowl. Add the pork and mix well. Cover and refrigerate for several hours or overnight.

Preheat the oven to 350°F. Drain the pork and reserve the marinade. Add the pork to a nonstick pan and cook until browned all over. Transfer to an ovenproof dish and bake 30 minutes. Slice diagonally.

Heat the oil in a wok, add the onion, carrot, and zucchini, and stir-fry over high heat until tender. Blend the cornstarch with the reserved marinade and a little water and add to the wok. Add the snow peas and bean sprouts and cook, stirring until sauce boils and thickens. Serve with the pork. If you want, serve with 2 tablespoons cooked brown rice (adds 70 calories).

Quick and Easy

Five-Minute Breakfasts

Scrambled Eggs Three Ways

Tomato and Chive

200 CALORIES   SERVES 1

Take 2 small eggs and whisk together in a bowl with a pinch of salt and plenty of black pepper. Heat a pat of butter in a pan and add the eggs. Use a spatula to push the eggs around the pan for 30 seconds to 1 minute until cooked to your liking. Stir in a sprinkle of snipped chives and serve on a couple of thick slices cut from a beefsteak tomato.

Creamy Smoked Salmon

310 CALORIES   SERVES 1

Whisk 1 tablespoon crème fraîche with 2 eggs. Melt 1 teaspoon butter in a skillet and pour in the egg mixture. Cook, stirring, until the eggs are halfway done. Add a sprinkle of chives and 2 ounces diced smoked salmon, then cook until eggs are done.

Chili Cheese

230 CALORIES   SERVES 1

Scramble 2 eggs with ½ teaspoon finely chopped chile. When the eggs are halfway done, add a handful of grated Parmesan and continue cooking until done to your liking.

Cottage Cheese Three Ways

Pear and Walnuts

210 CALORIES   SERVES 1

Spoon 3½ ounces cottage cheese into a bowl. Core and dice a small pear and stir into the cheese. Scatter on a handful of chopped walnuts.

Middle Eastern

90 CALORIES   SERVES 1

Spoon 3½ ounces cottage cheese into a bowl. Finely chop 1 tomato, a 2-inch piece of cucumber, and a handful of flat-leaf parsley. Stir into the cheese, add a squeeze of lemon juice, and season with black pepper.

Raspberry and Spinach

140 CALORIES   SERVES 1

Spoon 3½ ounces cottage cheese into a bowl. Coarsely chop a handful of baby spinach and stir into the cheese. Top with a handful of raspberries.

Avocado Three Ways

Poached Egg

200 CALORIES   SERVES 1

Scoop out the flesh from half an avocado and cut into thick slices. Sprinkle with a pinch of paprika. Poach an egg, place on top of the avocado, and season well.

Edam and Pecans

320 CALORIES   SERVES 1

Scoop out the flesh from half an avocado and dice. Place in a bowl and add a matchbox-sized piece of Edam cheese, diced, and a handful of pecans.

Tuna and Scallions

200 CALORIES   SERVES 1

Scoop out the flesh from half an avocado and place in a bowl. Add a small can of tuna in water, drained, and a squeeze of lemon juice. Mash together and stir in a chopped scallion. Serve on slices of beefsteak tomato.

No-Fuss Lunches

Mediterranean Platter

220 CALORIES   SERVES 1

Mix 2 tablespoons prepared hummus, a matchbox-sized piece of feta, a small handful of olives, 2 to 3 anchovies, 1 chopped red bell pepper, a 3-inch piece of cucumber cut into sticks, and a handful of halved cherry tomatoes.

Mexican Platter

350 CALORIES   SERVES 1

Mix 2 tablespoons each of prepared guacamole, salsa, and sour cream, 3½ ounces cooked chicken strips, and serve with 1 carrot and 1 celery stalk cut into dipping sticks.

No-Carb Ploughman's Lunch

290 CALORIES   SERVES 1

On a plate, place 1 apple, cored and cut into thick slices, with 2 stalks of celery, a matchbox-sized piece of cheddar, 2 slices of ham, a handful of walnuts, and a dollop of chutney (look for a low-sugar option).

Cheesy Baked Beans

260 CALORIES   SERVES 1

Season 2 portobello mushrooms and place under the broiler for 2 minutes. Heat half a can of baked beans in a pan, add a splash of Worcestershire sauce, and melt in a handful of grated mozzarella. Serve on the mushrooms.

Peanut Butter Dip

230 CALORIES   SERVES 1

Place 2 tablespoons peanut butter in a bowl, add 1 tablespoon soft cheese, and mix well. Cut 1 celery stalk, 1 carrot, a 3-inch piece of cucumber, and 1 red bell pepper into sticks to dip.

Sardine Dip

320 CALORIES   SERVES 1

Place 2 tablespoons soft cheese in a bowl and add a small can of drained sardines and a squeeze of lemon juice. Season with plenty of black pepper and mix well. Cut 1 celery stalk, 1 carrot, a 3-inch piece of cucumber, and 1 red bell pepper into sticks to dip.

Simple Suppers

Five Ways to Jazz Up a Chicken Breast

Lime and Ginger

130 CALORIES   SERVES 1

Mix the juice of ½ lime with ½ teaspoon five-spice powder, a drizzle of olive oil, a splash of fish sauce, and 1 teaspoon ginger paste. Mix together and pour over the chicken. Panfry or bake.

Almond and Basil

190 CALORIES   SERVES 1

Finely chop a handful of basil and place in a bowl with 1 tablespoon ground almonds and 1 tablespoon grated Parmesan. Season with salt and black pepper, drizzle in a little olive oil, and mix together. Spoon over the chicken and bake.

Pepper and Olive

170 CALORIES   SERVES 1

Finely chop 2 red bell peppers. Mix with a handful of finely chopped black olives and a pinch of crushed red pepper flakes. Spoon over the chicken with a drizzle of olive oil and bake.

Basil and Pine Nut

220 CALORIES   SERVES 1

Place a handful of basil in a food processor and add 1 tablespoon pine nuts, 1 tablespoon grated Parmesan, salt and black pepper, and a drizzle of olive oil and process to make a pesto. Spoon over the chicken and bake.

Spinach and Ricotta

230 CALORIES   SERVES 1

Finely chop a handful of spinach leaves. Place 2 tablespoons ricotta in a bowl, stir in the spinach, and add 1 tablespoon pine nuts. Make a slit lengthways along the side of the chicken and spoon the ricotta mixture into the middle. Drizzle with olive oil, season with salt and black pepper, and bake.

Three Ways to Jazz Up a Salmon Steak

Soy Sauce and Scallion

240 CALORIES   SERVES 1

Mix the juice of a lemon with 1 tablespoon each soy sauce and oyster sauce, 1 teaspoon grated ginger, and a chopped scallion. Rub the mixture over a salmon steak and place in the refrigerator to marinate for 1 hour or overnight. When ready to cook, drain the fish and panfry, adding the remaining marinade for the last few minutes.

Lime and Coriander

200 CALORIES   SERVES 1

Use a mortar and pestle to crush a handful of cilantro leaves into the juice of a lime. Mix in ½ teaspoon ground cumin and a pinch of red pepper flakes. Cover the salmon with the cilantro mixture and panfry or bake.

Spicy Sesame Seed Crust

250 CALORIES   SERVES 1

Mix 1 tablespoon sesame seeds with a pinch of cayenne pepper and a squeeze of lemon juice. Place a salmon steak under the broiler and cook on one side. Turn, spoon on the sesame seed mixture, and broil on the other side.

Three Ways to Jazz Up a Lamb Chop

Mint

170 CALORIES   SERVES 1

Use a mortar and pestle to crush a handful of mint with 1 tablespoon lemon juice and 1 tablespoon balsamic vinegar. Serve with a grilled lamb chop.

Mustard

180 CALORIES   SERVES 1

Crush 1 garlic clove and mix with 2 teaspoons Dijon mustard and a handful of chopped rosemary leaves. Spread over a lamb chop before cooking.

Pecan Crunch

220 CALORIES   SERVES 1

Mix a handful of pecans with 2 teaspoons lemongrass paste and 1 handful each of chopped thyme and flat-leaf parsley. Gently crush and spread on the lamb before cooking.

Three Ways with Zucchini Ribbons

Making the Ribbons

20 CALORIES   SERVES 1

Allow 1 zucchini per person. Use a spiralizer or a vegetable peeler to make the zucchini ribbons. Heat a skillet with a drizzle of olive oil and cook the ribbons for 2 to 3 minutes, until softened. Season with a pinch of salt and plenty of black pepper. Serve with any of the following sauces.

Bolognese

260 CALORIES   SERVES 4

Heat a drizzle of olive oil in a large pan and add 1 teaspoon Italian seasoning, a chopped red onion, a diced celery stalk, and a diced carrot; sauté for 10 minutes. Add 14 ounces lean ground beef and cook until evenly brown. Add 14 ounces of canned chopped tomatoes, 1 tablespoon each tomato puree and Worcestershire sauce, and season well with a pinch of salt and plenty of black pepper. Bring to a boil, stir well, reduce the heat to a simmer, cover, and cook for 1 to 1½ hours.

Salmon and Crème Fraîche

330 CALORIES   SERVES 1

Mix 2 to 3 tablespoons crème fraîche with 2 ounces cooked flaked salmon and 2 tablespoons cooked frozen peas. Heat gently in a saucepan.

Arrabiata

150 CALORIES   SERVES 3

Heat a drizzle of olive oil in a pan, add 1 teaspoon each dried oregano and thyme, 1 chopped garlic clove, 1 to 2 crushed fresh chiles, and the chopped stems from a handful of basil. Fry for few minutes. Add 14 ounces of canned chopped tomatoes and 1 tablespoon tomato puree. Simmer uncovered for about 8 minutes to let the excess water evaporate. Reduce the heat and cook for another few minutes, stirring occasionally. Add 1 tablespoon balsamic vinegar, a pinch of salt, black pepper to taste, and then stir in a handful of torn basil.

Three Ways with Cauliflower "Rice"

Making the Cauliflower "Rice"

30 CALORIES   SERVES 4

Cut the hard core and stalks from 1 head cauliflower and pulse the rest in a food processor to make grains the size of rice. Then either place into a heatproof bowl, cover with plastic wrap, pierce, and microwave for 7 minutes on high (there is no need to add any water) or spread the cauliflower grains thinly on a baking tray and bake in a medium oven for 10 to 15 minutes. Stir in some chopped cilantro or toasted cumin seeds for flavor. Serve with any of the following.

Vegetable Curry

270 CALORIES   SERVES 3

Heat a drizzle of oil in a large pan, add a chopped red onion, and cook for 8 minutes, until softened. Add a diced zucchini, a chopped red bell pepper, 3½ ounces chopped mushrooms, and 1 small peeled and diced butternut squash; mix in 2 to 3 tablespoons curry paste of your choice and 14 ounces of canned chopped tomatoes and bring to a boil. Reduce the heat and simmer for 25 to 30 minutes, adding a splash of water as needed.

Chicken and Pea "Pilaf"

170 CALORIES   SERVES 1

Heat a drizzle of oil in a pan and add 3½ ounces cooked chopped chicken and 2 tablespoons cooked frozen peas. Cook until the peas soften and then mix in the cauliflower rice.

Mushroom "Risotto"

210 CALORIES   SERVES 1

Sauté 3½ ounces chopped mushrooms in a drizzle of olive oil and a tiny bit of butter. Add some chopped rosemary leaves and 1½ ounces diced goat cheese and then mix in the cauliflower rice.

Three Quick Soups

Miso with Baby Vegetables

70 CALORIES   SERVES 1

Prepare the miso soup from a packet according to the directions and add 2 handfuls of baby vegetables, such as baby corn, sugar snap peas, and snow peas.

Pho with Cooked Chicken and Spinach

130 CALORIES   SERVES 1

Prepare a pho base from a packet and add 3½ ounces cooked chicken and 2 large handfuls baby spinach.

Consommé with Celeriac and Scallion

40 CALORIES   SERVES 1

Prepare the consommé from a packet and add 2 chopped scallions and 3 ounces grated celeriac.

Guilt-Free Baking

Zucchini and Pumpkin Seed Muffins

170 CALORIES   SERVES 12

> 3 tablespoons butter
> 1 zucchini
> 1 apple, cored
> Juice of 1 orange
> 4 large eggs
> 5 ounces coconut flour
> 1 teaspoon baking powder
> 1 teaspoon mixed spice (pumpkin pie spice)
> 2 ounces pumpkin seeds

Preheat the oven to 425°F. Line the cups of a muffin pan with paper liners.

Melt the butter in a small pan and set aside. Grate the zucchini and apple into a bowl. Beat the egg and then stir into the grated zucchini and apple. Add the orange juice and melted butter and stir well.

Sift the flour, baking powder, and mixed spice into a separate bowl and gradually stir the wet mixture into the dry mixture until sticky and well combined. Stir in the pumpkin seeds.

Divide the mixture among the muffin cups. Bake for 12 to 15 minutes, or until a skewer inserted into the center of the muffins comes out clean.

Cheesy Scones

180 CALORIES   MAKES 12

> 6¼ ounces coconut flour
> 6 tablespoons butter
> 6 eggs
> 1 teaspoon baking soda
> Pinch of salt
> 3 ounces cheddar, grated

Preheat the oven to 400°F and line a baking sheet with parchment paper. Combine all the ingredients in a food processor and pulse until blended. Allow the mixture to sit for 1 to 2 minutes. Form into 12 evenly sized patties and press onto the baking tray. Bake for 15 minutes, until golden.

Guilt-Free Brownies

120 CALORIES   MAKES 16

> 4 tablespoons coconut oil, melted
> 3½ ounces almond flour
> Pinch of salt
> ½ teaspoon baking powder
> 3½ ounces cacao nibs
> 6 dates
> 3 large eggs

Preheat the oven to 350°F and, using a little of the coconut oil, grease an 8-inch square baking pan. Mix all the ingredients together, transfer to the baking pan, and smooth over with a spatula. Bake for 20 minutes.

Appendix

The Different Types of Diabetes

Type 1 diabetes is also known as "early onset" because it typically occurs in childhood, though it can occur later in life. For various reasons the body stops producing insulin, and so type 1 diabetics have to get insulin by injection or via a pump. Although this type of diabetes is not closely linked to weight gain, keeping weight down and remaining active are still important.

Type 2 diabetes is by far the most common form (90 percent) and typically used to occur after the age of forty, though now it is starting to appear earlier and earlier. It happens when you become severely insulin resistant or your pancreas stops producing enough insulin. There are many causes, but high levels of fat in the liver and pancreas seem to be particularly important.

Gestational diabetes affects pregnant women. No one really knows why it happens, but one theory is that hormones produced during pregnancy can block insulin receptors, making some women more insulin-resistant. It is important to test for this condition because it can affect the long-term health of mother and child. Babies who are exposed to high levels of glucose in the womb are more likely to become obese and develop diabetes later in life. In most women the insulin resistance disappears soon after the child is born, but an Australian study found that 25 percent go on to develop diabetes within fifteen years.[53]

Further Blood Measurements

A1C Test

This is also known as the glycated hemoglobin or hemoglobin A1c test. Instead of measuring a single point in time (fasting glucose), this gives an estimate of your average blood sugar levels over the past few months.

Normal range: Below 6.0 percent (42 mmol/mol)
Prediabetes: 6.0–6.4 percent (42 to 47 mmol/mol)
Diabetic: Over 6.5 percent (42 to 47 mmol/mol)

Why is A1C important? According to Diabetes UK, "People with diabetes who reduce their A1C by less than 1 percent can cut their risk of dying within 5 years by 50 percent."

The Glucose Tolerance Test

This is a measure of how well your body is able to handle a big hit of sugar. After overnight fasting you have a blood test and are given a sugary drink, then a series of blood tests over the next two hours. Initially your blood sugar will spike. At the end of two hours, however, it should have fallen back below 7.8 mmol/l. If not, you have problems.

Prediabetic (impaired glucose tolerance):   7.9 to 11 mmol/l
Diabetic: Over 11.0 mmol/L

In pregnant women it is a concern if the 2-hour level is above 7.9 mmol/l because of the increased risks for the baby.

This book contains everything you need to know to do the 8-Week Blood Sugar Diet. But if you would like more information, advice, or support, please go to www.thebloodsugardiet.com.

This site is in its early days, and we would greatly appreciate feedback. We want to help build a community where people share experiences and recipes and support each other through the difficult times. It will include the latest research and up-to-date advice for professionals and dieters alike.

Acknowledgments

This book would not have been possible without the many scientists who gave so generously of their time and their research, most notably Dr. Roy Taylor. I am also indebted to those former diabetics who shared their experiences of being on the diet. Finally, a huge thanks to Rebecca Nicolson, Aurea Carpenter, the Short Books team, and the team at Atria, for their hard work and their support through the years.

Notes

1 Arch Mainhous III et al. Prevalence of prediabetes in England from 2003 to 2011. *British Medical Journal.* June 2014. http://bmjopen.bmj.com/content/4/6/e005002.full.

2 Xu Y et al. Prevalence and control of diabetes in Chinese adults. *JAMA.* September 2013. http://www.ncbi.nlm.nih.gov/pubmed/24002281.

3 Lee Gross et al. Increased consumption of refined carbohydrates and the epidemic of type 2 diabetes in the US. *American Journal of Clinical Nutrition.* 2004. http://ajcn.nutrition.org/content/79/5/774.full.

4 The Look Ahead Research Group. Cardiovascular effects of intensive lifestyle intervention in type 2 diabetes. *New England Journal of Medicine.* 2013. http://www.nejm.org/doi/full/10.1056/NEJMoa1212914.

5 David Ludwig and Mark Friedman. Always hungry? Here's why. *New York Times.* May 16, 2014. http://www.nytimes.com/2014/05/18/opinion/sunday/always-hungry-heres-why.html.

6 David Ludwig. Effects of diet on metabolism in humans. Presentation at Culinary Institute of America. 2012. David Ludwig et al. High glycemic foods, overeating, and obesity. *Pediatrics.* 1999. 103:E26.

7 Ludwig. Effects of diet on metabolism in humans.

8 E. L. Barr et al. Risk of cardiovascular and all-cause mortality in individuals with diabetes mellitus, impaired fasting glucose, and impaired glucose tolerance. *Circulation.* July 10, 2007. http://www.ncbi.nlm.nih.gov/pubmed/17576864.

9 T. Ohara et al. Glucose tolerance status and risk of dementia in the community. *Neurology.* September 2011. http://www.neurology.org/content/77/12/1126.abstract.

10 Looking older: the effect of higher blood sugar levels. Leiden University Medical Center. http://www.research.leiden.edu/news/looking-older-blood-sugar-plays-a-role.html.

11 W. J. Pories et al. Who would have thought it? *Annals of Surgery,* http://www.ncbi.nlm.nih.gov/pmc/articles/PMC1234815.

12 Roy Taylor. Type 2 diabetes: etiology and reversibility. *Diabetes Care.* 2013. http://care.diabetesjournals.org/content/36/4/1047.short.

13 R. Boussageon et al. Reappraisal of metformin efficacy in the treatment of Type 2 diabetes: a meta-analysis of randomized controlled trials. *PLOS Medicine.* April 10, 2012. http://journals.plos.org/plos medicine/article?id=10.1371/journal.pmed.1001204.

14 E. L. Lim. Reversal of Type 2 diabetes: normalization of beta cell function in association with decreased pancreas and liver triacylglycerol. *Diabetologia.* 2011. http://www.ncbi.nlm.nih.gov/pubmed /21656330.

15 S. Steven et al. Restoring normoglycaemia by use of a very low calorie diet. *Diabetic Medicine.* 2015. http://www.ncbi.nlm.nih.gov/pubmed /25683066.

16 Richard Surwit. *The Mind-Body Diabetes Revolution.* Da Capo Press. 2005. Page 29.

17 Ibid.

18 E. Donga et al. A single night of partial sleep deprivation induces insulin resistance in multiple metabolic pathways in healthy subjects. *Journal of Clinical Endocrinology & Metabolism.* 2010;95(6):2963–8. http://www.ncbi.nlm.nih.gov/pubmed/20371664

19 O. Ajala et al. Systematic review and meta-analysis of different dietary approaches to the management of Type 2 diabetes. *American Journal of Clinical Nutrition.* 2013. http://www.ncbi.nlm.nih.gov/ pubmed/23364002.

20 D. Unwin and J. Unwin. Low carbohydrate diet to achieve weight loss and improve A1C in Type 2 diabetes and prediabetes: experience from one general practice. *Practical Diabetes.* 2014. http://www .abc.net.au/catalyst/extras/low&20carb/Low&20Carb&20Diet&20f or&20Weight&20Loss&20and&20Diabetes&20-&20Unwin&202014 .pdf.

21 Myths, presumptions, and facts about obesity. *New England Journal of Medicine.* 2013. http://www.nejm.org/doi/full/10.1056/ NEJMsa1208051.

22 K. Purcell. The effect of rate of weight loss on long term weight management: a randomized controlled trial. *Lancet/Diabetes & Endocrinology.* 2014. http://www.thelancet.com/journals/landia/article/ PIIS2213-8587(14)70200-1/abstract.

23 A. Keys et al. *The Minnesota starvation experiment.* University of Minnesota. 1944. http://www.apa.org/monitor/2013/10/hunger.aspx.

24 C. Zauner et al. Resting energy expenditure in short-term starvation is increased as a result of an increase in serum norepinephrine. *American Journal of Clinical Nutrition.* 2000. http://ajcn.nutrition.org/content/71/6/1511.full.

25 Myths, presumptions, and facts about obesity, *New England Journal of Medicine.* 2013. http://www.nejm.org/doi/full/10.1056/NEJMsa1208051.

26 R. Estruch et al. Primary prevention of cardiovascular disease with a Mediterranean diet. *New England Journal of Medicine.* 2013. http://www.nejm.org/doi/full/10.1056/NEJMoa1200303#t=articleMethod.

27 R. Gotink et al. Standardized mindfulness-based interventions in healthcare: an overview of systematic reviews and meta-analyses of RCTs. *PLOS One.* 2015. http://journals.plos.org/plosone/article?id=10.1371/journal.pone.0124344.

28 R. Estruch et al. Primary prevention of cardiovascular disease with a Mediterranean diet. *New England Journal of Medicine.* 2013. http://www.nejm.org/doi/full/10.1056/NEJMoa1200303#t=articleMethods.

29 M. Kratz et al. The relationship between high-fat dairy consumption and obesity, cardiovascular, and metabolic disease. *European Journal of Nutrition.* 2012. http://link.springer.com/article/10.1007%2Fs00394-012-0418-1.

30 American College of Cardiology. Mediterranean diet may lower risk of diabetes. 2014. http://www.sciencedaily.com/releases/2014/03/140327100806.htm.

31 E. Toledo et al. Mediterranean diet and invasive breast cancer risk among women at high cardiovascular risk. *JAMA.* 2015. http://archinte.jamanetwork.com/article.aspx?articleid=2434738&resultClick=.

32 E. Martinez-Lapiscina et al. Mediterranean diet improves cognition. *Journal of Neurology, Neurosurgery & Psychiatry.* 2013. http://jnnp.bmj.com/content/84/12/1318.

33 Y. Gepner et al. Effects of initiating moderate alcohol intake on cardiometabolic risk in adults with Type 2 diabetes. *Annals of Internal Medicine.* 2015. http://annals.org/article.aspx?articleid=2456121.

34 N. Harkin et al. Diet and the prevention of cardiovascular disease: physicians' knowledge, attitudes and practice. *Journal of American College of Cardiology.* 2015. http://content.onlinejacc.org/article.aspx?articleid=2198773.

35 Low-fat diet not a cure-all. *JAMA.* http://www.hsph.harvard.edu/nutritionsource/low-fat.

36 E. Ford et al. Trends in mean waist circumference and abdominal obesity among US adults, 1999–2012. http://jama.jamanetwork.com /article.aspx?articleid=1904816.

37 Diabetes Prevention Program (DPP). http://www.niddk.nih.gov/ about-niddk/research-areas/diabetes/diabetes-prevention-program-dpp/Pages/default.aspx.

38 E. L. Lim. Reversal of Type 2 diabetes: normalisation of beta cell function in association with decreased pancreas and liver triacyl-glycerol. *Diabetologia*. 2011. http://www.ncbi.nlm.nih.gov/pubmed /21656330.

39 S. Steven et al. Restoring normoglycaemia by use of a very low calorie diet. *Diabetic Medicine*. 2015. http://www.ncbi.nlm.nih.gov/ pubmed/25683066.

40 D. Neal et al. The pull of the past: when do habits persist despite conflict with motives? USC. 2011. http://www.feinberg.northwestern .edu/sites/ipham/docs/WW_WIP20130122_Habits.pdf.

41 B. Wansink et al. Slim by design: kitchen counter correlates of obesity. Cornell University, SSRN. 2015.

42 E. Helander et al. Are breaks in self-weighing associated with weight gain? *PLOS One*. 2014. http://journals.plos.org/plosone/article?id= 10.1371/journal.pone.0113164.

43 M. Harvie et al. The effect of intermittent energy and carbohydrate restriction v. daily energy restriction on weight loss and metabolic disease risk markers in overweight women. *British Journal of Nutrition*. 2013. http://www.ncbi.nlm.nih.gov/pubmed/23591120.

44 R. Ross. Does exercise without weight loss improve insulin sensitivity? *Diabetes Care*. 2003.

45 Coronary heart disease and physical activity of work. *Lancet*. 265(1953):1053–1057.

46 E. G. Wilmot et al. Sedentary time in adults and the association with diabetes, cardiovascular disease and death: systematic review and meta-analysis. *Diabetologia*. August 14, 2012.

47 J. Veerman et al. Television viewing time and reduced life expectancy: a life table analysis. *British Journal of Sports Medicine*. 2012. http://www.ncbi.nlm.nih.gov/pubmed/23007179.

48 M. C. Peddie et al. Interrupting prolonged sitting impacts blood sugar metabolism. *American Journal of Clinical Nutrition*. 2013. http://www .cpmedical.net/newsletter/interrupting-prolonged-sitting-impacts-blood-sugar-metabolism.

49 J. Buckley et al. Standing-based office work shows encouraging signs of attenuating post-prandial glycaemic excursion. University of Chester. 2013. http://oem.bmj.com/content/early/2013/12/02/oemed-2013-101823.full.pdf?keytype=ref&ijkey=fvcEm117fzTcT51.

50 The effects of free-living interval-walking training on glycemic control, body composition, and physical fitness in Type 2 diabetic patients: a randomized, controlled trial. *Diabetes Care.* 2013. http://www.ncbi.nlm.nih.gov/pubmed/23002086.

51 B. Klika et al. High-intensity circuit training using bodyweight. *ACSM'S Health & Fitness Journal.* May/June 2013. http://journals.lww.com/acsm-healthfitness/fulltext/2013/05000/high_intensity_circuit_training_using_body_weight_.5.aspx.

52 Neural correlates of mindfulness meditation-related anxiety relief. *SCAN.* June 2013. http://scan.oxfordjournals.org/content/early/2013/06/03/scan.nst041.full.pdf.

53 A. J. Leet et al. Gestational diabetes mellitus: clinical predictors and long-term risk of developing type 2 diabetes: a retrospective cohort study using survival analysis. *Diabetes Care.* 2007. http://www.ncbi.nlm.nih.gov/pubmed/17392549.

Index

A

A1C test, 228
activity, 93, 227
    aerobic, 152
    stairs and, 136, 147
    standing and, 93, 143–46, 148
    see also exercise
adrenaline, 24, 60
aerobic activity, 152
aging, 31
alcohol, 98–99, 101, 121, 134
Alzheimer's disease, 31
American Diabetes Association,
    108
American Heart Association, 19, 20
American Journal of Clinical
    Nutrition, 19
amino acids, 81
amputation, 28–29, 32, 42, 57,
    65–66
arteries, 20, 30

B

bariatric surgery, *see* weight loss
    surgery

BBC Television, 6, 7
Beattie, Colin, 45–47
belt, wearing, 135
blindness, 30, 32
blood, fat in, 9
blood pressure, 34
    high, *see* hypertension
blood sugar, 8, 28–29
    checking, 107, 111, 139–40
    emotions and, 60
    exercise and, *see* exercise
    liver and pancreas and, 39
    raised, *see* raised blood sugar
    spikes in, 72, 73–74, 79
Blood Sugar Diet, 79, 91–113
    buddy or group for, 111
    clearing out cupboards
        before, 109–10
    core principles of, 91–95
    diary for, 105
    800 calories in, 46, 48, 50,
        51, 91, 115, 127, 138–39,
        140
    exercise and, *see* exercise
    goals in, 110–11

Blood Sugar Diet (*cont.*)
  with meal-replacement
    shakes, 50–51, 115–16
  medical checkups and, 139–40
  Mediterranean Diet and, *see*
    Mediterranean Diet
  in practice, 115–41
  preparation for, 102–12
  questions and answers on,
    118–22
  with real food, 50–51, 116, 117
  recipes for, *see* recipes
  talking to doctor before,
    103–4, 108
  tests to do before, *see* tests
  timeline for what to do
    and what to expect in,
    122–32
  weight gain in, 140–41
  when to start, 111–12
  see also very low-calorie diets
blood sugar monitoring kit, 107,
  111
Blood Sugar Way of Life, 126,
  132–37
blood vessels, 29–30
BMI, 55, 106, 111
Boston Children's Hospital, 24
brain:
  dementia and, 30–31, 32, 98
  Mediterranean diet and, 98
  mental fuzziness and, 26
  mindfulness and, 161

breakfast, 24–25, 120
  recipes for, 170–76, 213–15
breakfast cereals, 100, 134
breast cancer, 98
breathing exercise, 161
British Medical Journal, 8, 44
brunch recipes, 177–81
Buckley, John, 145, 146

C
calories, 18, 20, 38
  body fat and, 23
  LPL and, 37
  in reduced-fat products, 21
  standing and, 146
  very low-calorie diets, *see*
    very low-calorie diets
cancer, 98, 102
Cannon, Walter, 60
carbohydrates, 72–75, 100, 118–19
  calories in, 20
  complex, unrefined, 73
  glycemic index and, 73–75
  glycemic load and, 24, 74–75
  insulin and, 22–25, 73
  low-carb diets, *see* low-carb
    diets
  quiz on your relationship to,
    69–72
  refined, easily digestible, 19,
    22, 23–24, 65, 72–73, 79
  rise in consumption of, 19–22
  see also sugar

Cassie, 11, 57–60, 158
catastrophic thinking, 158–59
Centers for Disease Control
    (CDC), 8, 9
Cervantes, Carlos, 51–54, 157
children:
    diabetes in, 18
    overweight, 24
cholesterol, 8, 9, 32, 99
collagen, 31, 82
Confucius, 102
Cornell University, 134
cortisol, 60, 94, 157
cravings, 137
cupboards, 109–10, 134–35

D

dairy, low-fat vs. high-fat, 97–98
death, 30
    life expectancy, 42, 57
de La Monte, Suzanne, 31
dementia, 30–31, 32, 98
depression, 61, 62, 63
diabesity (diabetes plus obesity),
    6, 10, 19, 76, 165
diabetes, 104
    gestational, 57, 227–28
    type 1, 18, 104, 227
    type 2, *see* type 2 diabetes
Diabetes Care, 162
Diabetes UK, 2, 48
diary, 105
diet buddy, 111

diet products, 21, 133, 165
diets, 6
    crash, 80, 84–85
    5:2 approach in, 7, 127,
        138–39, 140
    Last Chance, 80–82
    low-carb, *see* low-carb diets
    low-fat, *see* low-fat diets
    Mediterranean, *see*
        Mediterranean Diet
    myths about, 10–11
    6:1 approach in, 140
    very low-calorie, *see* very
        low-calorie diets
dining out, 136
dinner recipes, 195–212
    simple, 217–23
DiReCT (Diabetes Remission
    Clinical Trial), 51
doctor, 103–4
    checkups with, 139–40
    tests to ask about, 108
dog, walking, 137
Doughty, Richard, 129
dual-energy X-ray absorptiometry
    (DEXA) scan, 108–9

E

Eat, Fast, Live Longer, 7
eating:
    comfort, 94
    habits of, 133
eggs, 24–25, 100

Eisenhower, Dwight D., 19
elastin, 31
emotions, 60–61
ethnicity, 55
exercise, 37, 93–94, 143–56
    high-intensity training, 152–56
    strength training, 86, 93–94,
        150–52
    walking, 37–38, 93, 145,
        146–50, 152
eyes, 30, 32
    retinopathy in, 103

F
family, 109–10, 111
FastDiet, The (Mosley and
    Spencer), 7, 139
fasting, 79
    anxieties about, 50
    each week, 137
    intermittent, 7, 137, 139
    metabolic rate and, 85–86
fat, body:
    belt and, 135
    in blood, 9
    BMI and, 55, 106, 111
    calories and, 23
    heart and, 38
    insulin and, 22–23, 24, 38
    in liver, 1, 38–39, 47, 48, 76,
        92, 111, 165, 227
    location of, 28, 36–38
    obesity, *see* obesity

    in pancreas, 1, 38–39, 47, 48,
        111, 165, 227
    personal threshold for, 9–10,
        39, 111
    subcutaneous, 38
    TOFIs (thin on the outside,
        fat on the inside) and, 38
    visceral (abdominal), 9, 38–39,
        91–92, 106–7, 153, 165
fat, dietary, 19, 165
    calories in, 20
    healthful, 101, 102
    heart disease and, 19–21,
        99–102
    low-fat diets, *see* low-fat diets
    oils, 98, 101
    reduced-fat products, 21
    saturated, 19, 20
    war on, 19–22
Fat Chance (Lustig), 23
FDA, 81
fiber, 19, 73, 76–77
fight-or-flight response, 60
Finer, Nick, 83–84
5:2 diet, 7, 138–39, 140
Fixing Dad, 62
food:
    in cupboards, 109–10, 134–35
    diary of, 105
    shopping for, 136
France, 20
Friedman, Mark, 23–24
friends, 111

fructose, 75–76
fruit, 75, 76, 101, 119–20

G
Gadde, Kishore, 83
gestational diabetes, 57, 227–28
Gill, Jason, 37
Glasgow University, 37, 51
glucose, 75
    drugs for lowering, 50
    fasting, measuring, 107–8
    tolerance test, 228–29
glycemic index (GI), 73–75
glycemic load (GL), 24, 74–75
glycogen, 153
goals, 110–11
    weight loss, 86, 110–11
good things, acknowledging, 137
grocery shopping, 136
gut bacteria, 76–77
gut hormones, 36

H
Hanks, Tom, 9
Harvard School of Public
    Health, 102
Headspace, 160
Health and Fitness Journal, 150
heart, fat around, 38
heart attacks, 30, 32, 42, 97, 144
heart disease, 19, 34–35, 144
    fat consumption and, 19–21,
        99–102

heart rate (pulse), 106
Helicobacter pylori, 43
Hemingway, Ernest, 145
high blood sugar, *see* raised
    blood sugar
high-intensity training (HIT),
    152–56
hobbies, 137
Hollingsworth, Kieran, 47
hormones:
    gut, 36
    insulin, *see* insulin
    PYY, 133
    stress, *see* stress hormones
Hu, Frank, 107
hunger, 43, 48, 59, 79, 86, 122,
    137
    feeling full, 119, 133
hypertension, 9, 32
    medication for, 50, 103

I
impaired glucose tolerance, *see*
    prediabetes
impotence, 30, 32
insulin, 8, 36, 227
    body fat and, 22–23, 24, 38
    carbohydrates and, 22–25, 73
    high blood sugar and, 22
    liver and pancreas and, 39
    LPL and, 36
    measuring levels of, 108
    medical, 35, 43, 103, 227

insulin (*cont.*)
  obesity and, 23
  stress and, 61, 157
insulin resistance, 9, 22, 93, 94,
  143, 227
  sleep deprivation and, 63–64
insulin resistance syndrome, *see*
  metabolic syndrome
insurance, 42
intermittent fasting, 7, 137, 139

J
Jacobson, Edmund, 162
Japan, 20, 31

K
Keys, Ancel, 19–20
kidney disease, 32
kitchen and cupboards, 109–10,
  134–35
Kratz, Mario, 97–98

L
LaBelle, Patti, 8–9
Last Chance Diet, 80–82
Lean, Mike, 51, 84
Leiden University, 31
Leonardo da Vinci, 145
Linn, Robert, 80–81
lipoprotein lipase (LPL), 36–37
life expectancy, 42, 57
liver:
  disease in, 38

fat in, 1, 38–39, 47, 48, 76,
  92, 111, 165, 227
fructose and, 75–76
stress hormones and, 61, 157
ultrasound scan of, 109
Look Ahead trial, 20–21
looks, 31
low-carb diets, 65–77, 117, 127
  see also Blood Sugar Diet;
    very low-calorie diets
low-fat diets, 6, 8, 20, 65, 119, 165
  and heart disease and stroke,
    19–21, 99–102
  success rate of, 20–21
Ludwig, David, 23–24, 25
lunch, soup, and salad recipes,
  182–95
  no-fuss lunches, 215–16
  quick soups, 223
Lustig, Robert, 23

M
magnetic resonance imaging
  (MRI), 109
Marshall, Barry, 43–44
Martin, Corby, 83
Mattson, Mark, 7
Maudsley, Henry, 60
Mayer, Jean, 21
meal-replacement shakes,
  50–51, 115–16
meals:
  dining out and, 136

eating habits and, 133
medications, 103
  blood pressure, 50, 103
  glucose-lowering, 50
medications for diabetes, 10,
    42–45, 103
  insulin, 35, 43, 103, 227
  metformin, 42–43, 103
Mediterranean Diet, 66–67,
    92–93, 95–102, 117, 127
  scoring your current diet, 96–97
  what to eat, 100–101
mental fuzziness, 26
metabolic rate, 85–86
metabolic syndrome, 9
  see also insulin resistance
metformin, 42–43, 103
mindfulness, 94–95, 159–63
Monroe, Marilyn, 107
muscle relaxation exercise, 162–63
muscles, 22, 23, 37, 81

N
National Institute for Health
    and Care Excellence, 108
National Institutes of Health, 122
Newcastle University, 2, 33, 104
New England Journal of Medicine,
    82, 96
New York Times, 23
Nobel Prize for Medicine, 44
nonalcoholic fatty liver disease
    (NAFLD), 38

Norman, Lorna, 39–41
nuts, 101, 102, 120–21

O
oatmeal, 24, 100
obesity:
  in children, 24
  diabesity, 6, 10, 19, 76, 165
  diabetes and, 28
  epidemic of, 17–32
  insulin and, 23
  see also fat, body
olive oil, 98, 101, 102
omelets, 24
ovaries, polycystic, 59

P
pancreas, 22, 143, 227
  fat in, 1, 38–39, 47, 48, 111,
    165, 227
  stress hormones and, 61
photographing yourself, 107
polycystic ovaries, 59
polyphenols, 98
Pories, Walter, 34
prediabetes, 5
  Blood Sugar Diet and, 121–22
  metabolic syndrome and, 9
  reversing, *see* reversal of type
    2 diabetes or prediabetes
  statistics on, 8, 9
  weight loss surgery and, 35
  see also raised blood sugar

PREDIMED trial, 95–97
pregnancy, 104, 229
    gestational diabetes and, 57,
        227–28
progressive muscle relaxation,
    162–63
Prolinn, 81–82
protein, 19, 81, 101
    calories in, 20
Puddicombe, Andy, 160
pulse, 106
Purcell, Katrina, 83
PYY, 133

R
raised blood sugar, 10
    blood vessels and, 29–30
    brain and, 30–31
    effects of, 5, 29–31
    fat location and, 28
    insulin and, 22
    looks and, 31
    spikes, 72, 73–74, 79
    symptoms of, 5
    see also prediabetes
recipes, 167–225
    breakfasts, 170–76, 213–15
    brunches, 177–81
    guilt-free baking, 224–25
    lunches, 182–95, 215–16
    quick and easy, 213–23
    salads, 182–95
    soups, 182–95, 223

suppers, 195–212, 217–23
retinopathy, 103
reversal of type 2 diabetes or
        prediabetes, 2, 33–54
    with very low-calorie diet,
        10, 11, 33, 47–54
    after weight loss surgery, 1,
        34–36
risks for type 2 diabetes, 55–64
    quiz on, 56
    stress and, 60–61
Royal Free Hospital, 5

S
salad, soup, and lunch recipes,
        182–95
    no-fuss lunches, 215–16
    quick soups, 223
Schenker, Sarah, 117
sedentary lifestyle, 144
seeds, 121
Seligman, Martin, 137
sitting, 144–45
6:1 diet, 140
skin, 31
sleep, 26, 34, 99
    insulin resistance and, 63–64
Smietana, Bob, 25–27, 157–58
Smith, Will, 102
snacking, 135, 165
    on fruit, 119–20
Social Cognitive and Affective
        Neuroscience, 161

soup, 133–34
soup, salad, and lunch recipes, 182–95
   no-fuss lunches, 215–16
   quick soups, 223
Spencer, Mimi, 7
stairs, 136, 147
standing, 93, 143–46, 148
starvation mode, 85
steps, tracking, 105–6, 146–47
stomach ulcers, 43–44
strength training, 86, 93–94, 150–52
stress, 60–61, 157
stress hormones, 24, 60–61, 107, 157
   cortisol, 60, 94, 157
stress reduction, 94, 157–63
   mindfulness in, 94–95, 159–63
stroke, 21, 30, 32, 97, 99–102, 144
sugar, 8, 20, 22, 23, 65, 72, 100
   fiber and, 76
   fructose, 75–76
   glucose, *see* glucose
   in reduced-fat products, 21
supper recipes, 195–212
   simple, 217–23
surgery:
   amputation, 28–29, 32, 42, 57, 65–66
   weight loss, *see* weight loss surgery

syndrome X, 9
   see also insulin resistance

T
Taylor, Roy, 11, 33–36, 38–39, 40, 45, 47–51, 53, 84, 104, 130–31
television watching, 144, 145
tests, 105–9
   A1C, 228
   fasting glucose, 107–8
   glucose tolerance, 228–29
   measuring pulse, weight, and waist, 106–7
   specialist, 108–9
Timmons, Jamie, 152–53
TOFIs (thin on the outside, fat on the inside), 38
Truth About Exercise, The, 37
Truth About Personality, The, 94
type 1 diabetes, 18, 104, 227
type 2 diabetes, 227
   author's diagnosis of, 5, 6–7
   in children, 18
   confirming presence of, 104
   costs of, 42
   dementia and, 30–31
   as lifelong disease, 1
   medications for, *see* medications for diabetes
   obesity and, 28
   physical costs of, 32
   reversing, *see* reversal of type 2 diabetes or prediabetes

type 2 diabetes (*cont.*)
　　risks for, *see* risks for type 2
　　　diabetes
　　sedentary lifestyle and, 144

U
ulcers, 43–44
Ulcer Wars, 43, 44
University of Southern
　　California, 133
University of Sydney, 74
Unwin, David, 67–69

V
Varady, Krista, 7
vegetables, 101, 120
very low-calorie diets, 79–87
　　with meal-replacement
　　　shakes, 50–51, 115–16
　　hunger and, 86
　　Last Chance, 80–82
　　metabolic rate and, 85–86
　　myths about, 79, 83–84, 85–87
　　with real food, 50–51, 116,
　　　117
　　reversal of type 2 diabetes or
　　　prediabetes with, 10, 11,
　　　33, 47–54
　　water weight and, 80, 87
　　weight gain following, 79,
　　　83–84
　　see also Blood Sugar Diet
Vietnam, 55–57

W
waist size, 106–7
walking, 37–38, 93, 145, 146–50, 152
Warren, Robin, 43, 44
water intake, 87, 122
water weight, 80, 87
weaknesses, knowing, 135
weighing yourself, 106, 135
weight:
　　BMI and, 55, 106, 111
　　and risk of blood sugar
　　　problems, 55
　　type 1 diabetes and, 227
　　see also fat, body
weight loss:
　　goals for, 86, 110–11
　　gradual, 6, 80, 82, 83, 84
　　water in, 80, 87
weight loss, rapid, 84
　　myths about, 79, 83–84, 85–87
　　weight gain following, 79, 83–84
　　see also very low-calorie diets
weight loss surgery, 1, 34–36
　　dumping syndrome after, 35
Whitington, Geoff, 61–63, 157
wine, 99, 101, 121, 134
Women's Health Initiative
　　(WHI) Dietary Modifi-
　　cation Trial, 102
World Health Organization, 108

Y
yogurt, 100

Find even more life-changing tips for eating right and staying healthy in Dr. Mosley's *the FastDiet*, *FastExercise*, and the all-new compilation,

the FastLife!

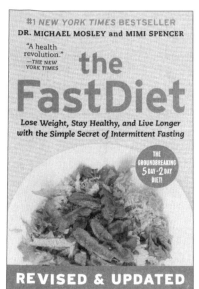

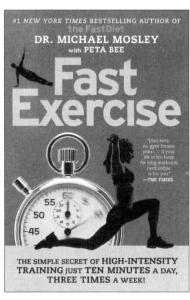

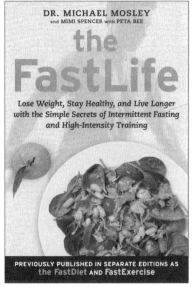